Women and Health

Women and Health:
Feminist Perspectives

Edited by

Sue Wilkinson and Celia Kitzinger

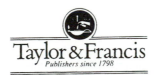

Taylor & Francis
Publishers since 1798

UK   Taylor & Francis Ltd, 4 John St., London WC1N 2ET
USA   Taylor & Francis Inc., 1900 Frost Road, Suite 101, Bristol, PA 19007

First published 1994

A Catalogue Record for this book is available from the British Library

ISBN 0 7484 0148 2 (cloth)
ISBN 0 7484 0149 0 (paper)

Library of Congress Cataloguing-in-Publication Data are available on request

Typeset in 10/13 pt CG Times Roman
by RGM Associates, Lord Street, Southport, England

Printed in Great Britain by Burgess Science Press, Basingstoke on paper which has a specified pH value on final paper manufacture of not less than 7.5 and is therefore 'acid free'.

Contents

Introduction

Feminist Perspectives on Women and Health

Sue Wilkinson and Celia Kitzinger

This book began life as a symposium at the 1992 Annual Conference of the British Psychological Society. Entitled 'Women and Health: Feminist Perspectives', this symposium was unusual in at least two respects. First, it included cutting-edge research originating within a variety of disciplines (including cross-disciplinary and multidisciplinary work), not just from within psychology; and, second, its focus was *feminist* research on health, rather than health research on women (Graham, 1993a).

Although there has been a recent upsurge of interest in women's health as a topic within psychology (e.g. Nicolson and Ussher, 1992; Niven and Carroll, 1993; Travis 1988a, 1988b) and sociology (e.g. Abbott and Payne, 1990; Miles, 1991; Stacey, 1988), most of this work has remained within the confines of disciplinary boundaries. Moreover, within psychology, very little of it has been conducted within a feminist framework. Perhaps for this reason, the 1992 symposium attracted a great deal of interest, and we were subsequently invited to guest-edit a Special Issue of *Health Psychology Update* (Wilkinson and Kitzinger, 1993), focusing on specifically feminist research on women's health. In so doing, we included contributions from researchers in and across a number of other disciplines, in order to exemplify the best of contemporary feminist research in the area.

As the project expanded and developed into an edited volume, these two features — a feminist focus and a multidisciplinary range of contributors — remained central to our selection of material. All of the contributors included here acknowledge gender-based inequities in women's experiences of health and health care, and address the need for social and political change.[1] This volume constitutes, we believe, the most important collection of feminist research on women's health since

Lewin and Olesen's (1985) *Women, Health and Healing*. It is more comprehensive than that volume (the research represented here spans the disciplines of psychology, sociology, social policy, social anthropology and economics), and also demonstrates the development of feminist theorising and activism in relation to health over the past decade.

Of course, the contributors to this book do not agree on definitions of feminism; nor do they identify the same key issues facing women in relation to health; nor do they advocate the same strategies for change. While recognising *external* resistance to change from organised medicine and other interest groups (see, for example, Meg Stacey's chapter in this volume; Walsh, 1977), the women's health movement is divided *internally* over inequities due to differences between women (including 'race', class, sexual identity, age and (dis)ability), and the specific priorities and forms of intervention these require. In this volume, we have not addressed such differences as discrete categories,[2] but have asked our contributors to weave considerations of difference throughout their chapters.

Mindful of major national differences in historical and political context between western industrialized countries, and, particularly between British and North American feminist campaigns on health-related issues (see Lewin and Olesen, 1985, pp. 3–7), we invited only British contributors to this volume. We asked contributors to reflect on cross-Atlantic, and broader international, differences (see, in particular, Doyal, this volume) wherever appropriate; however, such reflections come from a British perspective on these issues. We do not even begin to address the task of major cross-cultural comparison, nor do we survey the issues relating to women and development, although there is a growing literature in these areas: e.g. Jacobson, 1990, 1991; Koblinsky *et al.*, 1993; Whelehan, 1988.

In contrast to a number of books on women's health (e.g. Roberts, 1978, 1992; Graham, 1984), we have not placed any special emphasis on women's traditional, particularly reproductive, roles — the chapters by Wiles and Spallone are the exceptions.[3] Rather, the eleven chapters included here consider the issues surrounding women's health and wellbeing across a broad range of activities and different stages of the lifespan.

The first and last chapters 'frame' the more specific considerations of particular health issues with a general analysis of the operation of male power in organised medicine — a theme which also threads through a number of other chapters. Ellen Goudsmit's opening chapter considers the ways in which women's health problems have often been trivialized or dismissed by — mostly male — health care practitioners as 'all in the mind', while Meg Stacey draws on her personal experience as a member of the General Medical Council to expose the ways in which one of the statutory bodies of British medicine creates and maintains its deeply patriarchal power base. In both analyses, the actual experiences of women — as medical 'consumers' or as Council members — are shown to be conspicuously absent.

The remaining chapters are organised — loosely — on a 'lifespan' basis. Chapters two, three and four deal, respectively, with early (hetero)sexual experiences, pregnancy and body image, and the impact of reproductive technologies. Rachel Thomson and Janet Holland look at young women's practice — or otherwise — of 'safer' (hetero)sex in the context of gendered power relations, and offer suggestions for services and education in sexual health which are more appropriate to women's needs. Rose Wiles's chapter reports a study of 'fat' women's feelings about changes in their weight and body image during and after pregnancy. Most of these women reported feeling more satisfied with themselves and more socially acceptable during pregnancy, and Wiles locates these findings within the context of the prevailing ideal-ized/sexualized images of femininity produced by men, and accepted by the majority of women. The formal operation of male power is the focus again in Pat Spallone's contribution. She examines how scientific priorities shape the medical development of new reproductive technologies, largely ignoring the specificities of women's bodies, and promoting the ideology of the heterosexual nuclear family, with scant assessment of the long-term health risks entailed.

The next three chapters look, broadly, at work and at activities construed by some women as 'leisure'. Lesley Doyal provides a broad overview of the relationship between work outside the home and women's health, focusing on the physical and psychological hazards which reflect sexual divisions both in the structure and organisation of waged work and in the wider society. Elizabeth Ettorre's and Hilary Graham's chapters both consider women's use of substances. Ettorre provides a feminist critique of much traditional work on substance use (including food, alcohol, cigarettes, tranquillisers and other drugs), and Graham focuses specifically on the relationship between gender divisions, poverty and smoking. Drawing on women's own reported experiences of smoking, she considers the extent to which this 'habit' may offer an antidote to the boredom, isolation and stress that can accompany full-time caring for young children on a low income.

Chapters eight, nine and ten are concerned with illness and social change in mid to late life, examining, respectively, breast cancer, the menopause and hormone replacement 'therapy', and bereavement. In chapter eight, based on our own work, we return again to male power in organised medicine and the media, together with the 'psychologising' messages of the self-help literature for women with breast cancer. We argue that these are all distressing — and potentially harmful — to the breast cancer sufferer, and offer some suggestions for developing a feminist approach to breast cancer. Kate Hunt continues the analysis of male medical power in chapter nine, looking at the social construction of the menopause and the increasing use of hormone replacement 'therapy'. Again, we see prevailing images of 'ideal' femininity and narrowly-prescribed roles for women, and, as with reproductive technologies, poor assessment of long-term health risks. Based on her interviews with women who have been widowed, in chapter ten Jane Littlewood argues that not only is the experience of widowhood poorly understood, and largely consigned to the 'private' sphere, but that social policy provision for widows operates actively to reinforce women's subordinate position in society.

Together, these eleven chapters provide a broad sample of contemporary British feminist work on women and health. Ranging from theoretical analyses and review chapters to reports of empirical research (both qualitative and quantitative), they demonstrate the range and diversity of current feminist research on women's health. The shared aim of all the contributors is to understand and improve the health and health care of women across the lifespan.

Notes

1 For introductory reviews of such inequities and related feminist activism, see, for example, Hockey, 1993; Ruzek, 1986; for more sustained analyses see, for example, Doyal, 1979, 1994; Graham, 1984, 1993b.
2 See, in contrast, the growing literature on, for example, lesbian health — e.g. *Health Care for Women International*, 1992; Hepburn and Gutierrez, 1988 — or black women's health — e.g. Ahmad, 1993; White, 1990.
3 Again there is, of course, a substantial body of feminist work focusing exclusively on reproduction and reproductive technologies: e.g. Katz Rothman, 1989; Kitzinger, 1978; Klein, 1989; Phoenix *et al.*, 1991; Rowland, 1992; Spallone, 1992; and also on domestic work, including 'caring' in its broadest sense: e.g. Dalley, 1988; Finch and Groves, 1983; Oakley, 1984; Ungerson, 1987, 1990.

References

ABBOTT, P. and PAYNE, S. (1990) *New Directions in the Sociology of Health*, London, Falmer.

AHMAD, W.I.U. (Ed.) (1993) *'Race' and Health in Contemporary Britain*, Buckingham, Open University Press.

DALLEY, G. (1988) *Ideologies of Caring: Rethinking Community and Collectivism*, London, Macmillan.

DOYAL, L. (1979) *The Political Economy of Health*, London, Pluto.

DOYAL, L. (1994) *What Makes Women Sick? Gender and the Politics of Health*, London, Macmillan.

FINCH, J. and GROVES, D. (1983) *A Labour of Love: Women, Work and Caring*, London, Routledge.

GRAHAM, H. (1984) *Women, Health and the Family*, Brighton, Wheatsheaf.

GRAHAM, H. (1993a) 'Research Literatures on Women and Health', in WILKINSON, S. and KITZINGER, C. (Eds) Special Issue of *Health Psychology Update, Women and Health: Feminist Perspectives*, 12.

GRAHAM, H. (1993b) *Hardship and Health in Women's Lives*, Hemel Hempstead, Harvester-Wheatsheaf.

Health Care for Women International, Special Issue: Lesbian Health: What are the Issues? (1992) 13(2).

HEPBURN, C. and GUTIERREZ, B. (1988) *Alive and Well: A Lesbian Health Guide*, Freedom, CA, The Crossing Press.

HOCKEY, J. (1993) 'Women and Health', in RICHARDSON, D. and ROBINSON, V. (Eds) *Introducing Women's Studies: Feminist Theory and Practice*, London, Macmillan.

JACOBSON, J.L. (1990) *The Global Politics of Abortion*, Worldwatch Paper 97, Washington DC, Worldwatch Institute.

JACOBSON, J.L. (1991) *Women's Reproductive Health: The Silent Emergency*, Worldwatch Paper 102, Washington DC, Worldwatch Institute.

KATZ ROTHMAN, B. (1989) *Recreating Motherhood: Ideology and Technology in a Patriarchal Society*, New York, W.W. Norton.

KITZINGER, S. (1978) *Women as Mothers*, London, Fontana.

KLEIN, R. (1989) *Infertility: Women Speak Out about their Experiences of Reproductive Medicine*, London, Pandora.

KOBLINSKY, M., TIMYANN and GAY, J. (1993) (Eds) *The Health of Women: A Global Perspective*, Boulder, CO: Westview Press.

LEWIN, E. and OLESEN, V. (1985) *Women, Health and Healing: Toward a New Perspective*, London, Tavistock.

MILES, A. (1991) *Women, Health and Medicine*, Milton Keynes, Open University Press.

NICOLSON, P. and USSHER, J. (1992) *The Psychology of Women's Health and Health Care*, London, Macmillan.

NIVEN, C. and CARROLL, D. (1993) *The Health Psychology of Women*, Basel, Harwood Academic.

OAKLEY, A. (1984) *The Sociology of Housework*, Second Edition, Oxford, Blackwell.

PHOENIX, A., WOOLLETT, A. and LLOYD, E. (Eds) (1981) *Motherhood: Meanings, Practices and Ideologies*, London, Sage.

ROBERTS, H. (1978) *Women, Health and Reproduction*, London, Routledge.

ROBERTS, H. (1992) *Women's Health Matters*, London, Routledge.

ROWLAND, R. (1992) *Living Laboratories*, London, Lime Tree.

RUZEK, S. (1986) 'Feminist Visions of Health: An International Perspective', in MITCHELL, J. and OAKLEY, A. (Eds) *What Is Feminism?* Oxford, Blackwell.

SPALLONE, P. (1992) *Generation Games*, London, The Women's Press.
STACEY, M. (1988) *The Sociology of Health and Healing*, London, Unwin Hyman.
TRAVIS, C.B. (1988a) *Women and Health Psychology: Biomedical Issues*, Hillsdale, NJ, Erlbaum.
TRAVIS, C.B. (1988b) *Women and Health Psychology: Mental Health Issues*, Hillsdale, NJ, Erlbaum.
UNGERSON, C. (1987) *Policy is Personal: Sex, Gender and Informal Care*, London, Tavistock.
UNGERSON, C. (Ed.) (1990) *Gender and Caring*, Hemel Hempstead, Harvester-Wheatsheaf.
WALSH, MARY ROTH (1977) *Doctors Wanted: No Women Need Apply: Sexual Barriers in the Medical Profession, 1835–1975*, New Haven and London, Yale University Press.
WHELEHAN, P. (Ed.) (1988) *Women and Health: Cross Cultural Perspectives*, Massachusetts, Bergin and Garvey.
WHITE, E. (1990) *The Black Women's Health Book*, Seattle, The Seal Press.
WILKINSON, S. and KITZINGER, C. (Eds) (1993) Special Issue of *Health Psychology Update, Women and Health: Feminist Perspectives*, 12.

Chapter 1

All in Her Mind! Stereotypic Views and the Psychologisation of Women's Illness

Ellen M. Goudsmit

Psychologisation is the term used to describe the emphasis on psychological factors in illness where there is little or no evidence to justify it. In many cases, it reflects a lack of knowledge and/or a shortage of resources (Goudsmit and Gadd, 1991). However, research has also indicated that a practitioner's assessment may be unduly influenced by the patient's gender. In this chapter, I will summarise the main ways in which stereotypic views of women can act as a source of bias both in the evaluation of symptoms, and in the choice of treatment.

First of all, let me illustrate the problem of psychologisation with two examples. A few years ago, the *British Medical Journal* carried a report about three women who were admitted to casualty suffering from breathlessness and panic symptoms (Treasure *et al.*, 1987). The diagnosis made was hysterical hyperventilation — two were referred to the psychiatrist and the third was sent home with a prescription for diazepam. Within three days, however, all were re-admitted, in various states of consciousness. This time, a more thorough investigation was done and this revealed that their symptoms were actually due to diabetes. According to the authors, the assumption that the problem was psychological had led to the omission of a physical examination and put three people's lives at risk. To put it another way, the doctors concerned had jumped to conclusions and had not checked that their diagnosis was correct. This is a fairly typical case of psychologisation and clearly shows how dangerous it can be.

Another example was reported more recently by consultant haematologist Milica Brozovic (1989). It concerns a woman who changed to a job which 'proved to be rather difficult'. She became anxious and tired, and three months into her new job, she also developed intermittent cramp-like pain. Her GP diagnosed irritable bowel syndrome (IBS), precipitated by the stress of the job, and advised that she take a short period of sick leave. However, the pain did not subside and although she consulted her GP on several more occasions, and she went to her local casualty unit, no one challenged this diagnosis. In fact, there were a number of cues which were inconsistent with IBS but these were continually overlooked. When she was examined by Brozovic, she noted an easily palpable mass in the left iliac fossa and an emergency operation later confirmed cancer of the sigmoid colon.

The Weak Woman

Although the literature shows that men are not immune, it is noteworthy that the vast majority of case-histories of psychologisation feature female patients. While some may argue that this is just coincidence, there is also good evidence that being a woman does influence many practitioners' clinical judgement. Looking back over some of the older literature, one can see that women were often portrayed as weak, suggestible, emotionally unbalanced, irrational, manipulative, and unable to cope with even relatively minor stress.

For instance, authors writing about dysmenorrhoea (period pains) commented about its prevalence in 'highly strung' and 'nervous' women, and how a 'faulty outlook' could lead to the exaggeration of minor discomfort (cf Lennane and Lennane, 1973). Similarly, premenstrual syndrome was dismissed as 'discomfort' which all women should be able to cope with, without medical intervention. In both these conditions, accounts of the illnesses often included references to the literature on somatisation, implying that certain women exaggerate their distress, perhaps to escape responsibility and effort (e.g. Notman, 1982). What the articles don't mention is the possibility that recurring unpleasant symptoms, like pain and nausea, can undermine a woman's self-confidence and self-esteem and that this could also account for the raised scores on psychometric tests (Goudsmit, 1988). The literature simply didn't, and still doesn't, acknowledge the fact that emotional problems may often be the result, rather than the cause of certain conditions (Lennane and Lennane, 1973).

While some of the disorders above are characterized by common symptoms like tiredness, tension and pain, all of which may be due to a variety of problems including stress, psychologisation has also been documented in conditions where symptoms are much more specific. For example, women complaining of mastalgia (severe breast pain) have been described as 'frustrated, unhappy nulliparae' and 'irritable and suggestive' (cf Preece *et al.*, 1978), the implication being that these factors may have played an important role in the development of the disease. Interestingly, when women with mastalgia were given psychometric tests, their scores were very similar to those of women with varicose veins and lower than those of psychiatric patients. The condition is now thought to be mainly due to hormonal factors (Brush, personal communication).

Infection or Hysteria?

Another example of how stereotypes of women can colour people's thinking is the story of the epidemic at the Royal Free Hospital in 1955 (Crowley *et al.*, 1957; Ramsay 1988). This outbreak of a two-phased infection closed the hospital for a while, and affected more than 200 members of staff. Most of them were nurses; 90 per cent of them were women. Fifteen years after the event, two young male psychiatrists were given access to some incomplete reports and the notes of those who were *not* thought to have had Royal Free disease (McEvedy and Beard, 1970a). Instead of restricting their conclusions to that group, they implied that the whole outbreak had been due to mass hysteria. Their reasoning was that: (1) the illness affected primarily young, segregated women; (2) some of the symptoms are commonly seen in anxiety and hyperventilation; (3) no infective agent was identified; and (4) the outbreak was therefore mass hysteria.

In reaching this conclusion, they dismissed important clinical findings including the involvement of the immune system. They also assumed that the nurses were segregated, which was later questioned. However, what was really interesting about this episode, and what is often not realised, is that the epidemic wasn't limited to the main hospital. The first cases occurred at the Royal Free, but it spread quickly to other hospitals in North London. Amongst these was a hospital and a nursing home run for and by women. It occurred to me that if the epidemic had been the result of fear and anxiety amongst suggestible women, one would have expected these *female-only* institutions to have been at the top of the list of hospitals affected. However, only the Eastman Dental Hospital had *fewer* cases (Crowley *et al.*, 1957).

Many researchers now believe that the culprit was an enterovirus (Hyde *et al.*, 1992) but for nearly twenty years, the mass hysteria explanation dominated the literature and the thinking about myalgic encephalomyelitis (M. E.). In contrast, a similar epidemic which affected a whole barrack of male soldiers was not classed as mass hysteria, and neither were all the epidemics which affected an equal number of men and women (McEvedy and Beard 1970b), even though they were by all accounts very similar conditions.

Aside from the examples documented in the clinic and in the literature, one can also find evidence of stereotypic views in academic institutions like medical schools. For instance, a report by Mary Howell (1974) includes a comment from a female student that: 'Women's illnesses are assumed psychosomatic until proven otherwise'. Another student revealed: 'Often women are portrayed as hysterical or as nagging mothers or as having trivial complaints. Men are almost never pointed to as having a psychological component to their illnesses — this is generally attributed to women'. Howell also notes how mothers are seen as 'complaining', and older women are 'demanding and bitchy'. According to Brozovic (1989), such attitudes are still around.

Different Sex, Different Treatment

The tendency of some doctors to think that women exaggerate their distress and their assumption that psychological factors play a major role in their illness may explain why symptoms reported by women are investigated less thoroughly than the same symptoms in men. For example, a small study by Armitage *et al.* (1979) discovered that physicians ordered more extensive tests and procedures for men than for women with the same complaint. Discussing the possibility that male doctors take illness more seriously in men than in women, they suggested that the physicians 'might have been responding to current stereotypes that regard the male as typically stoic and the female as typically hypochondriacal'.

Two recent reports indicate that this gender bias still exists. Ayanian and Epstein (1991) studied patients hospitalised for coronary heart disease and found that women underwent fewer diagnostic and therapeutic procedures than men. A second study supported this, noting that women with cardiac disease were offered fewer procedures like coronary by-pass surgery than men, even though the women were more disabled and those procedures could have lessened the symptoms (Steingart *et al.*, 1991). The authors stated that the symptoms of chest pain in women were more likely to be attributed to non-cardiac causes. However, they did not expand on this.

Aside from stereotypic beliefs, what may have influenced a few of the practitioners is the way some women present their problems (Gillespie, 1988). If a patient is emotional, it could be interpreted as a sign of a more vulnerable, sensitive personality who may be prone to psychosomatic disorders. This is perfectly reasonable. However, the *assumption* that the cause is psychological or psychosomatic tends to stop many practitioners from checking for other contributory factors, and this may lead to errors. It is, therefore, important that physicians should assess all possible sources of a particular complaint and not just assume that an existing psychological disorder or stressful situation is responsible for all the existing symptoms.

In conclusion, the overemphasis of psychological factors in illness can lead to diagnostic errors, to inappropriate treatment, and to a great deal of unnecessary suffering. For these reasons, I would like to encourage all those concerned to take a more critical look at the evidence for psychological explanations, and to challenge existing sex-role stereotypes in medical schools, in clinical practice and most of all, in the medical literature.

References

ARMITAGE, K. J., SCHNEIDERMAN, L. J. and BASS, R. A. (1979) 'Response of physicians to medical complaints in men and women', *Journal of the American Medical Association*, **241**(20), 2186–2187.

AYANIAN, J. Z. and EPSTEIN, A. M. (1991) 'Differences in the use of procedures between women and men hospitalized for coronary heart disease', *New England Journal of Medicine*, **325**, 221–225.

BROZOVIC, M. (1989) 'With women in mind', *British Medical Journal*, **299**, 689.

CROWLEY, N., NELSON, M. and STOVIN, S. (1957) 'Epidemiological aspects of an outbreak of encephalomyelitis at the Royal Free Hospital in the Summer of 1955', *Journal of Hygiene*, **55**, 102–122.

GILLESPIE, L. (1988) *You Don't Have To Live With Cystitis*, London, Century.

GOUDSMIT, E. M. (1988) 'Psychological aspects of premenstrual symptoms', in BRUSH, M. G. and GOUDSMIT, E. M. (Eds) *Functional Disorders of the Menstrual Cycle*, Chichester, Wiley & Sons.

GOUDSMIT, E. M. and GADD, R. (1991) 'All in the mind? The psychologisation of illness', *The Psychologist*, **4**, 449–453.

HOWELL, M. C. (1974) 'What medical schools teach about women', *New England Journal of Medicine*, **291**, 304–307.

HYDE, B. M., GOLDSTEIN, J. and LEVINE, P. (Eds) (1992) *The Clinical and Scientific Basis of Myalgic Encephalomyelitis/Chronic Fatigue Syndrome*, Ottawa, Nightingale Research Foundation.

LENNANE, K. J. and LENNANE, R. J. (1973) 'Alleged psychogenic disorders in women — a possible manifestation of sexual prejudice', *New England Journal of Medicine*, **288**, 288–292.

McEvedy, C.P. and Beard, A.W. (1970a) 'The Royal Free epidemic of 1955: a reconsideration', *British Medical Journal*, **1**, 7–11.

McEvedy, C.P. and Beard, A.W. (1970b) 'Concept of benign myalgic encephalomyelitis', *British Medical Journal*, **1**, 11–15.

Notman, M. (1982) 'The psychiatrist's approach', in Debrovner, C.H. (Ed.) *Premenstrual Tension. A Multidisciplinary Approach*, New York, Human Science Press.

Preece, P.E., Mansel, R.E. and Hughes, L.E. (1978) 'Mastalgia: psychoneurosis or organic disease?', *British Medical Journal*, **1**, 29–30.

Ramsay, A.M. (1988) *Myalgic Encephalomyelitis and Postviral Fatigue States*, Second Edition, London, Gower Medical Publishing.

Steingart, R., Packer, M., Hamm, P., Coglianese, M.E., Gersh, B. *et al.* (1991) 'Sex differences in the management of coronary heart disease', *New England Journal of Medicine*, **325**, 226–230.

Treasure, R.A.R., Fowler, P.B.S., Millington, H.T. and Wise, P.H. (1987) 'Misdiagnosis of diabetic ketoacidosis as hyperventilation syndrome', *British Medical Journal*, **294**, 630.

Chapter 2

Young Women and Safer (Hetero)Sex: Context, Constraints and Strategies

Rachel Thomson and Janet Holland

Levels of teenage pregnancy and unprotected sex in the United Kingdom are among the highest in the developed world (Jones *et al.*, 1985). Statistically, unprotected sex is a 'normal' part of the sexual careers of heterosexual British adolescents (Bury, 1984; Wight, 1990). But what lies behind such statistics?

In this chapter we present some of the findings of the Women Risk and AIDS Project (WRAP),[1] illustrating the context and constraints that shape the practice of both unprotected and 'safer' sex. We will consider the practice of safer sex from the perspective of young heterosexual women. Our discussion falls into three parts: first, we consider the context within which young women become sexually active; we then explore some of the constraints upon the effective practice of safer heterosex by young women and consider strategies employed by them to control their sexual encounters; and finally, we make some suggestions about sex and HIV/AIDS education in the light of our findings.

As in other studies of adolescent sexuality, we found high levels of unprotected sex: 45 per cent of the sexually active members of our interview sample had, at some point, had sex unprotected against pregnancy; 70 per cent had practised sex unprotected against HIV/AIDS or any other sexually transmitted disease; 14 per cent became pregnant, and 7 per cent had abortions. In the following pages, we will attempt to give a sense of how young women perceive and experience sexual practice and the factors that might promote or inhibit the practice of safer heterosexual sex.

The WRAP Study

The Women Risk and AIDS project is a qualitative investigation of the sexual knowledge, practices and meanings of 150 young women aged between sixteen and twenty-one in Manchester and London. We devised a purposive sample based on the variables of age (three age groups) ethnicity, sexual activity, and power, which was related to socio-economic class[2], education and work prospects. The power dimension was designed to address the degree of autonomy which young women might exercise in different areas of their life.

Overall in the sample we wanted a third of the young women to be sexually active and potentially at risk of contracting HIV; a third sexually active but not necessarily at risk (for example, in monogamous relationships as far as we (and they) know, and practising forms of safer sex); and a third not sexually active. In the event, 82 per cent of them were sexually active. We employed a pre-selection questionnaire covering a range of demographic variables, basic information on sexual knowledge and sex education, and on numbers and type of sexual relationships. These questionnaires could be filled in anonymously, or the young women could give a contact address so that we could, if appropriate, arrange for an interview. Some young women also agreed to keep diaries of their sexual behaviour and feelings for us.

The major method used in the study was an extensive and intensive interview, tape recorded and transcribed onto a computer and analysed with the aid of a qualitative programme called the Ethnograph. The interviews were semi-structured, the interviewer aimed to be responsive to what the young woman wanted to say, enabling her to direct or order the account of her own particular 'story'. The subjects always covered in the course of the interview were: a detailed exploration of the nature and type of their relationships (sexual, family, friendship), the quality and sources of their sex education, their knowledge of HIV and AIDS and the sources of that information. We discussed risk taking, safer sex, contraception, the double standard, trust, first sexual experiences, sexual practice and the negotiation of sexual encounters. Questions about their lifestyle, religion if relevant, their image of themselves and plans for the future were also included.

Context

The last twenty years has seen a significant increase in the incidence of teenage sexual activity, or more precisely in the incidence of teenage sexual intercourse. Surveys of sexual behaviour show that the age at which young people begin to have sexual intercourse has been falling since 1964 (Bury, 1984; Farrell, 1978; Ford and Bowie, 1988; Estaugh and Wheatley, 1990; Ford, 1993). See Table 2.1, adapted from Wight (1990). Recent research indicates that the dramatic fall in the age of first intercourse may have, in fact, taken place during the 1950s rather than in response to the availability of the pill, as previously supposed (Wellings *et al.*, 1994).

Table 2.1   Percentage of 16–18 year olds with experience of sexual intercourse by age, gender and year.

	1964*		1974/75**		1991***	
	Male	Female	Male	Female	Male	Female
16	14	5	32	21	53	51
17	26	10	50	37	67	67
18	34	17	65	47	83	83

*   An English sample from Bury, 1984;
**   An English and Welsh sample from Farrell, 1978;
*** A South West England sample from Ford, 1991.

Of the young women we interviewed, we found that 62 per cent were sexually active by, or at, age sixteen rising to 96 per cent by, or at, age twenty-one. We found that early sexual activity was slightly more likely among working class (wc) girls, the average age of first sex being 14.9 years as opposed to 16.3 years for middle class (mc) girls. Our data on average number of partners also varies slightly by class (see Table 2.2) with middle class respondents reporting a higher incidence of casual sex.

Table 2.2   (a) Average number of partners in WRAP sample.

	mc	wc	total
Age 16–17 years 11 months			
Casual with intercourse	1.31	0.42	0.7
Steady with intercourse	0.69	1.0	0.9
Age 18–19, 11			
Casual with intercourse	1.25	1.07	1.2
Steady with intercourse	1.63	1.0	1.3
Age 20–21, 11			
Casual with intercourse	6.81	3.39	5.02
Steady with intercourse	2.3	2.52	2.41
Overall average casual	3.3	1.7	
Overall average steady	1.7	1.6	

Table 2.2   (b) Average age first sex.

	mc	wc	total
Age 16–17, 11	15.07	13.57	14.07
Age 18–19, 11	16.08	14.71	15.57
Age 20–21, 11	17.23	15.59	16.27
Total	16.27	14.49	15.4

These figures should be treated with some caution as our in-depth qualitative data has shown the importance of cultural factors in the process by which young women define and name their sexual encounters. The social pressures against young heterosexual women defining a sexual encounter as 'casual' are very strong, and may be stronger within working class than middle class culture. Young women's own definitions of their sexual encounters are influenced by these factors; we found, for example, that the term 'steady relationship' was perceived primarily in terms of commitment rather than duration (see also Abrams *et al.*, 1990).

Learning about sex

It is important to understand that the context of sexual relationships for young women goes beyond empirical findings relating to the 'normal' level of sexual activity. As the previous observation about definitions of casual and steady relationships shows, before we can measure the incidence and indices of sexual behaviour, it is vital that we understand the way in which young women conceptualise their own and others' sexuality and sexual activity. The interviews we carried out with young women were concerned not only with the young women's sexual practice, but also with the meanings they attached to that practice. In order to understand these meanings it was necessary to enquire into the process by which young women learned about sex and sexuality, and within which their sexualities were socially constructed.

When we asked our interviewees where they learned about sex and sexuality we found that most of them had experienced almost no explicit discussion of sexual practice as such. There had been a great deal of discussion and interest around what we might call the rules of 'appropriate femininity'. School was one of the few places where any reference to the physicality of sex appeared, but this was in a selective, technical and scientific form. In general, these young women dismissed their school sex education as irrelevant to their concerns. The scientific language and approach was alienating, and the emphasis on reproduction and the natural world bore little relation to the pressures actually experienced by young women in relation to sex. As one put it 'what we learnt at school was nothing like real life'.

Significantly, the young women's accounts of school sex education were characterised by an absence of reference to physical sexuality or issues concerning sexual pleasure. In many cases, biological diagrams of male and female genitalia failed to include the clitoris, and references to non-reproductive aspects of sexual practice such as masturbation and homosexuality were far less frequent than those to periods, pregnancy, intercourse and STDs. Michelle Fine (1988) has documented a similar situation in relation to the educational ethos of American public school sex education where, she argues, a complete absence of discussion of sexuality and sexual pleasure in effect educates young women to ignore their sexual self interest.[3]

Discussion of the home as a source of sex education revealed that most of the communication about sex between parents (mainly mothers) and daughters takes place within a 'protective discourse', which although based on real fears for their daughter's welfare, passes on very negative images of sex and sexuality. Mothers are often keen to ensure that their daughters 'don't make the same mistakes' as they had themselves. The 'mistakes' mothers usually regretted centred on early pregnancy and the resulting limitation of their careers. Mothers rarely raised issues of sexual satisfaction or empowerment. In this context, sex is again firmly linked to the potential for reproduction, with mothers giving daughters contraception advice, against a backdrop of fear of active male sexuality. These warnings may well be necessary and realistic, but given in isolation they serve to reinforce the passive view of female sexuality which is implicit in school education. As Ros Coward notes, within such a discourse 'women's sexuality is limited to making a choice between yes and no' (Coward, 1984).

Female friends tended to be the most common source of information about sexual matters (see Table 2.3). Once again, we found that although contraceptive information was readily shared amongst friends there was very little discussion of sexual practice itself. This can be partially explained by the vulnerability felt by young heterosexual women in relation to their sexual reputation. The 'slag'/'drag' dichotomy (Lees, 1986, 1993) appears still to be very much a force (although often actively resisted), and has perhaps become more intractable with the relatively new addition of the label 'frigid' serving to restrict further young women's independent sexual development. In general, we found that young women used their female peer group or

Table 2.3   (a) Sources of sexual information (WRAP questionnaire sample).[1]

	parent	teachers	fem f	male f	mass m	books etc.
periods	**74**	32.9	59.7	2.6	12.9	38.5
hetero rels	44.2	30.8	**58.1**	30.0	33.3	33.7
homo rels	26.4	23.4	**43.1**	27.6	40.3	34.1
intercourse	43.3	43.3	**60.3**	33.9	26.8	38.3
contraception	41.3	45.6	**49.6**	16.9	0.2	46.0
pregnancy	**58.3**	48.4	49.6	10.3	25.2	39.9
abortion	31.7	38.1	**44.6**	9.1	0.2	38.9
masturbation	8.5	20.2	**38.7**	22.2	0.0	0.2
STD	28.6	45.6	37.5	17.5	39.1	**50.8**
AIDS	28.5	35.5	28.4	17.1	**57.7**	55.8

Table 2.3   (b) Perceived quality of sex education from three sources (interview sample).

	School		Home		Peers	
	N	%	N	%	N	%
Good	22	15	39	30	34	32
Adequate	31	22	30	23	44	42
Inadequate	88	61	61	47	18	17
Misleading	3	2	0	0	10	9
Totals	144	100	130	100	106	100

[1]Figures in **bold** indicate the source of information on that topic most frequently mentioned by the questionnaire sample.

best friend as a means of support and a space within which to discuss feelings and emotions, but rarely sex or desire. More explicit discussions of sexual practice including the only non-scientific language available to describe it was seen to be the domain of boys:

> But you know, fellas of my age, you'll hear them on the bus, 'oh I shagged her, I did this to her, I fucked her in this way'. I just look at them and think I bet you never.

> I remember there was lads that always sort of talked about it, it was always the lads, never the girls. You know, they'd say 'oh I wouldn't mind having her tonight', all this sort of thing. (Thomson and Scott, 1991).

Probably the most pervasive, if elusive, source of sex education for young women derives from the media and other forms of popular culture. These sources often carry contradictory messages, on one hand presenting undiluted images of romantic ideology, and on the other hand presenting male defined images of idealised femininity and sexual attractiveness. Although young women often acknowledged and resisted the sexist nature of many magazines and other forms of popular culture, the absence of other more positive sources of information made them reliant on these sources for information and guidance. In this way, romantic ideology and sexual knowledge inevitably became linked in the cultural framework within which the information is made available.

The cultural context within which young women learn about sex rarely offers or supports positive models of female sexuality. The available images tend to represent women as passive, as victims of male sexuality, and reproductive. The enduring dichotomy of the virgin and the whore works to discredit and distort expressions of female sexual agency. These ideologies militate against the development by young women of a sense of themselves as autonomous sexual beings, isolating young women from one another and alienating them from the practice of sexuality. Although frequently well versed on the mechanics of reproduction and the dangers of sexual activity, young women are ill equipped to confront these dangers since they have little conception of the nature of female sexual pleasure, and often no conception of female sexual self-interest. Sex is something which happens **to** them for the benefit of someone else. Sex can be a means to gain status in terms of a relationship ('being someone's girlfriend' or a mother can confer status) but sexual practice itself remains shrouded in mystery and silence. As such the context within which young women learn about sex and sexuality provides them with little verbal or conceptual ammunition with which to make informed and meaningful choices.

Constraints on the Practice of Safer Sex

Three major sets of constraints operate on young heterosexual women, rendering their possibilities for practising safer sex problematic. These are: the existing contraceptive culture, the symbolic meaning attached to condoms, and their own lack of power, autonomy and control within sexual situations.

Evidence from our research and that of others suggests that health education campaigns about safer sex and condom use have been effective in terms of the communication of information. In answer to the question 'what do you consider safe sex to be?' the young women responded almost without exception in terms of condom use. We also found that when asked 'would you be willing to ask a partner to use a condom in the future?' 77 per cent of our questionnaire sample answered yes, and only 7 per cent said no. But the qualitative data from the interviews revealed a rather more complex situation in which such good intentions were not necessarily borne out in practice, and where day-to-day fears of pregnancy far outweighed the apparently distant threat of HIV/AIDS. Only 23 per cent of the sexually active interviewees had **ever** used a condom as a prophylactic.

The gap between intention and practice, knowledge and behaviour, particularly acute in the case of young women, has been found by other researchers looking at young people and safer sex (Ford and Bowie, 1988; Ford and Morgan, 1989). Can young women be judged as immature, since they have the facts with which to make rational choices, and fail to do so? The accounts of sexual careers and encounters given to us by young heterosexual women suggest that the issue of condom use and safer sex is not merely one of informed choice and rational decision making, but cannot be understood without taking account of the **gendered** power relations which construct and constrain these choices and decisions (Holland *et al.*, 1994; Gavey, 1993; Waldby *et al.*, 1991).

Contraceptive Culture

The first constraint we draw attention to is that of the pre-existing contraceptive culture through which safer sex messages must be mediated. Before the widespread use of the pill, the contraceptive method most used by young people, discounting withdrawal, was the condom, and attitudes reflected this. Schofield found that most girls felt that contraception was a man's business (Schofield, 1965). During the late 1970s and 1980s, there was a major reversal in the responsibility for contraception as the pill became the preferred form (see Wight, 1990, p. 37) and the responsibility for contraception moved over more strongly to women, upon whom contraceptive services were increasingly targeted (Wight, 1990, p. 36–7). Recent research indicates that the reduction in the use of the pill amongst young people in the last few years, thought to be related to fears of cervical cancer and HIV, is now reversing, although there is conflicting evidence on this (*General Household Survey*, 1988; Schering Health Care, 1991). The pill remains the main form of contraception used by young women and it was certainly the most common form used by those who answered our questionnaire, being used by 24 per cent of them. The pill is not only seen as a reliable contraceptive, but its use does not intrude on the act of sexual intercourse. The use of a particular contraceptive can quite profoundly construct both the expectation and practice of sex. As Judith Bury has noted in a recent article 'the legacy of the last twenty years is that women are still assumed to be responsible for contraception yet, given the imbalance of power in sexual relationships, women may in practice have little effective control over safer sex' (Bury, 1991, p. 47).

Many of the young women to whom we spoke considered 'spontaneity' to be a central defining factor of sexual interaction. We have argued elsewhere (Holland *et al.*, 1990) that this emphasis on spontaneity in sex may in fact be a means of masking ignorance as well as serving effectively to remove agency on the part of young women. The ideology of appropriate femininity positions young heterosexual women as passive and unknowing sexual actors. To be knowledgeable about sex or to be seen to pursue sexual gratification is a sexual identity for which young women find little support. Many of the young women we spoke to expressed opposition to condom use for reasons related to this ideal of 'spontaneous' sex made possible by the pill where reproductive issues are rendered invisible. One young woman said:

> The climax to intercourse is all passion and kissing and I think to actually just stop and he puts a condom on, or me to turn around and say I want you to put this on, it just ruins the whole thing then.

The image of sex as spontaneous relates strongly both to romantic images of sex as being 'swept off one's feet', as it does to a lack of confidence about and knowledge of their own bodies. The 'rational' safer sex messages ('you know the risks, the choice is yours') can be seen as antithetical to an ideology of femininity which constructs sex as relinquishing control in the face of love.

Symbolic Meanings: Condoms, Romance and Trust

Responsibility for sexual safety as well as contraception means that young heterosexual women are faced with major contradictions in the context of sexual encounters, which can result in inconsistent outcomes. We found that condom use as contraceptive and prophylactic amongst our interviewees was often inconsistent. While 68 per cent of the sexually active young women had used condoms at least once as a contraceptive, only 20 per cent had used them regularly. As we have heard, 23 per cent had used condoms as a prophylactic, yet only 11.5 per cent had managed this consistently. Even in these cases, consistency could be related to small numbers of sexual encounters rather than efficacy of condom use.

Condoms are not neutral objects, but carry many symbolic meanings. They are associated with certain types of sex, significantly with sporadic sexual encounters, whether these are one night stands, early sexual experiences or sexual encounters outside an established relationship (Bury, 1984; Spencer, 1984; Day *et al.*, 1988; Nix *et al.*, 1988). There is a common sense assumption that negotiations about sex are easier in the context of a steady relationship, yet our data show[4] this is not necessarily the case. 'Going steady' implies a degree of trust which is lacking in less persistent sexual relationships. As a type of relationship, 'going steady' can be seen as a precursor of monogamy (whether serial or otherwise). The underlying moral code of monogamy calls for absolute trust despite the lack of actual security, particularly in terms of STDs and HIV infection. Trust, then, becomes a significant factor in decision making about condom use, and can in itself become a euphemism for monogamy.

While condom use characterises the early stages of a sexual relationship (if not the first sexual encounter in a relationship) we found that when a relationship was felt to be established, the young woman would cease condom use and transfer to the pill as a method of contraception. Continued condom use at this point would distinguish between its function as prophylactic and contraceptive at a time when the display of trust is considered to be crucial. This transition from condoms with a new partner to the pill with a steady partner is laden with symbolic meaning and can be used to signify the seriousness of a relationship, a way of demonstrating to a partner that he is special. As one of our respondents put it 'I went on the pill for him'. If condoms signify 'casual', 'illicit' or inexperienced sex, the pill is associated with grown up status and grown up sex. This makes the prospect of long term condom use highly problematic, as some of our respondents clearly indicated:

A: If you want to have relationships then you've got to trust them. Otherwise it's no good from the start. You have to believe what they tell you. You just hope they tell the truth. You can't find out if it's lies or not.

A: You've got to trust somebody at some time, you can't meet somebody and start, first time say, 'I know, let's use condoms I'm not on the pill' (even if you are) and then a

week later still be saying 'Let's use condoms' and a week
after that still be saying 'Let's use condoms' . . .

Q: You don't think you could do that long term?

A: You couldn't do that, no.

A: I'd like to think that I would want to use one [condom] but
I mean, you start off using one but are you going to carry
on using one every single time?

Yet we also found that there was a good deal of pressure on the young
women to define the relationship they were in as 'serious' (and therefore
steady) in order to justify sex within a model of appropriate femininity.
The question of what counts as a steady relationship is clouded by the
meanings associated with particular types of relationships, and by fears
for loss of reputation, particularly by the younger women. Most young
women are reluctant to describe themselves as having casual sex when
the culturally approved objective is to be in a steady, preferably
monogamous relationship. They are likely to expect or to express the
hope that relationships of short duration, including one night stands,
will in fact last. The positive associations of sex as leisure and pleasure
which can be found in gay and heterosexual male culture tend not to be
available to young heterosexual women. The tendency seems to be to
expect the relationship to last, relationships are 'steady' until proved
otherwise.

A: If I sleep with anyone I intend it to be a long term
relationship — so I don't know, because you don't like to
think of the end of a relationship when you start it.

Lack of Power, Autonomy and Control in Sexual Situations

The third constraint experienced by young women wishing to practice
safer heterosexual sex is the degree of control which they have within
sexual encounters. Power within sexual encounters should not merely be
defined in relation to the presence or absence of violence or its threat,
but pressure was present in the sexual encounters of a significant
minority of our sample. Thirty nine young women, 26 per cent of our
sample, indicated experiences in which men had exerted pressure on
them to have sexual intercourse. Of this 39, 13 had been raped and 10
had experienced sexual abuse as children. Ten of these 39 young women
had experienced more than one form of pressure on different occasions

(Holland *et al.*, 1992b). This group of the young women we interviewed **had** experienced some kind of sexual violence or pressure, but power is present within sexual relationships in some far less explicit but still crucial ways (Gavey, 1993). Many of the young women's objections to condom use centred around fears of partners' disapproval of condoms. Such disapproval was perceived to be related to issues of trust as mentioned above, but it was also related to ideas about male sexual pleasure and fears of its disruption.

The privileging of male sexual pleasure within our culture is experienced particularly strongly by young women who are unsure of their own sexual potential and agency. Requesting or insisting on condom use in this context can be a potentially subversive demand. The spontaneity of passion can be undermined by the recognition of risk and responsibility; sexual safety and sexual satisfaction pull against each other when the latter is defined in terms of men's fulfilment. We found that many of the young heterosexual women we interviewed experienced little pleasure in their sexual relationships, although we do have evidence to suggest that many gained a great deal of pleasure from non-penetrative sexual practice (see Ford, 1991). It seemed at times that what was valued was the social relationship with the partner rather than the sexual activity. Young women are not of course without the ability to choose and to act — but the full range of choices is rarely clear to them, and the social constraints within which they operate are severe. For a young woman to insist on the use of a condom for her own safety requires resisting the constraints and opposing the construction of sexual intercourse as a man's natural pleasure and a woman's natural duty (Holland *et al.*, 1994).

In our interview sample, 67 per cent of the sexually active young women had asked for condom use at some point in their sexual career. Of these, 21 per cent had asked and had been refused for varying reasons. Others had not even been able to ask, finding themselves muted by the contradictions of their situation, and despite their intentions were unable to initiate condom use. In very few cases were young men found to take responsibility in this area, and in these cases they were perceived to be exceptional by the young women concerned, who were surprised and pleased at their maturity and sense of responsibility.

A: I know I have been in situations where I haven't [used a condom]. I have simply thought to myself, well look, well. When I got pregnant, I thought to myself, 'I'm not using a condom here, I'm not using anything', but I just couldn't

say, just couldn't force myself to say, 'look you know' —
and then the consequences were disastrous. But at the time
I knew what I was doing, and I knew that I just couldn't
say it and knew that it was wrong.

A: About two weeks ago I ended up not asking him [to use a
condom] and had to go and get the morning after pill. I
wouldn't say anything, and kept thinking I'll say
something in a minute, it's just so difficult. I thought I'd
say something in a minute and then it was too late, and I
thought 'Oh no!' I didn't even know this person anyway.

Strategies

We have illustrated above some of the pressures which constrain young
women's capacity to ensure their own sexual safety. In this section we
will look at examples of ways in which some of the young women were
able to negotiate and enforce safer sex within their relationships. These
strategies have differing effectiveness, and we will conclude with some
comments on the potential for longer term strategies of education for
safer sex and practice within contraceptive services.

We found a number of strategies employed by young women in
order to manage to have safer sex:

- subterfuge
- avoiding vulnerability
- policing monogamy
- taking control

Subterfuge

A small number of the young women we interviewed reported adopting
a strategy for safer sex which entailed being on the pill but using its
invisibility as a cover to request condom use on the basis of fear of
pregnancy. In this way, problems associated with trust, with
appearances of sexual innocence and the taboo associated with the
prophylactic function of the condom could effectively be avoided in the
short term. The young women who used this strategy preferred it since it
did not place them in the position of having to challenge the gendered
power relations of the sexual encounter. But it is also a strategy which

challenges the romantic expectations of potential relationships and as such might be difficult to sustain consistently. It demands the acknowledgement of the transient nature of a sexual encounter. Not all young women are able to do this. This strategy becomes problematic if the relationship does in fact last.

Avoiding Vulnerability

Another latent strategy adopted by young women was the avoidance of vulnerability by establishing relationships with men who were younger and/or significantly less experienced or mature than themselves. This was usually not specifically in order to practice safer sex, but related to more general fears of vulnerability around sexuality and relationships.[5] These young women were particularly interesting as they seemed able to ensure that their own sexual needs were given status within their relationships. In most cases this included shared responsibility for and interest in sexual safety and contraception. Many of these young women expressed concern that they might not be able to negotiate the same relationship with future partners, particularly if that partner was sexually experienced themselves. One describes her relationship with a less experienced partner in this way:

> **A:** The bloke I am actually going out with is about three years younger than I am and we get on really well, and he hadn't actually had a sexual experience before that . . . so I was like the experienced one, although I had only done it about four or five times. So the way I used to ask questions, I used to love talking about it, and he was actually doing that, and it was just working it out ourselves. And because he had no sort of ideals about it, he was a lot more thoughtful of me which was why it is very different. Paul is the first bloke that I have actually said 'This is what I like to do', or 'Do it there, that's the wrong place'. And before I didn't really say nothing, and now I have actually demanded things or asked things, and said how I was feeling about things.

Policing Monogamy

Another group of young women who perceived themselves to be effectively 'safe' were those in monogamous relationships which they felt confident to actually be so. In a few cases, the young women had negotiated an HIV test before the relationship became sexual. In others, partners' sexual histories were known due to small and static social networks. Such strategies to a limited extent challenge the gendered morality of heterosexual culture by questioning the nature of trust. However, such a strategy does not necessarily affect actual sexual practice and partners remain vulnerable to the possibility of infidelity. It is a strategy which is dependent on having a certain type of relationship and not one to which everyone can or would want to ascribe. It is not a strategy which young women can take with them to new relationships.

Taking Control

A small number of the young women to whom we spoke had considered safer sex to be a more significant project. For them safer sex was seen as part of a wider reconsideration of their own sexual practice, pleasure and desire. They were young women who had reflected upon their sexual experiences and found them wanting in terms of their own agency and access to sexual pleasure. These young women considered safer sex to be more than condom use and considered the 'possibilities of non-penetrative sex' a means by which they could explore and privilege their own sexual needs. The safer sex repertoire of these young heterosexual women was considerably wider than those who perceived it simply to mean using a condom, and they were prepared to have to educate their partners about the validity and worth of a range of non-penetrative sexual practices. Such a strategy is effective precisely because it entails challenging a definition of sex structured by expectations of men's needs and desires and in doing so also challenges the implicit constraints to safer sex as mentioned above, spontaneity, loss of control, trusting to love and lack of self-esteem. While some of these young women excluded penetrative sex from their sexual practice others continued to enjoy it, but as one part of a wider sexual repertoire, using condoms when necessary. These young women experienced few if any problems negotiating condom use within this context. This strategy is not dependent on the context of the sexual encounter or relationship but can travel with the person from relationship to relationship. One empowered young woman described her understanding of safer sex and the means by which she employed these practices as follows:

> **A:** Safe sex is as pleasurable an experience as actual penetration. Oral sex, just things like touching somebody

else's body in a very gentle way. Kissing. Appreciating one another's bodies.

I think it's just as [much] fun, if not more. You concentrate on each other's needs a lot more, you're a lot more aware of them. You're aware of each other's bodies a lot more...Instead of 20 minutes of bang, bang bang, you've got a whole night; you watch the dawn come up and you're still there.

Q: Have you had to convert your partners? Have you come across men who understand sex as being more than penetration?

A: Yes...I've said, 'I don't want to do that', or 'why don't you try this?'. Before they know it they're converted, and they suddenly realise — 'well we haven't actually done it'. 'Well I'm tired now, haven't you had a good time?' You can change a lot of people's ideas.

But maintaining a sense of personal empowerment which is independent of context and relationship can be difficult and lonely.[6] It requires young women to negotiate a new model of sexuality which treats female sexual pleasure as a priority. Such a strategy has not as yet been taken seriously by the health education and mainstream family planning establishment (see also Wilton, 1991).

Some Thoughts on Implications for Practice and Conclusions

Many of the issues which we have identified in this chapter and the constraints on the practice of safer sex can only be approached through education. We have also noted, however, the limitations of the type of sex education offered by schools, and the way in which the conjunction of the scientific model of sex education offered by schools and the protective approach to sex education characteristic of the family can serve to educate young women against an awareness of sexual self interest. If sex education is to communicate effectively it needs to address the subject of sexuality as it affects young people themselves, including an awareness of the gendered power relations which structure sexual interaction and relationships.

We suggest that such programmes attempt to nurture and develop in young women a sense of self worth and self esteem and ally this to an awareness of their own sexual needs, desires and capacities, including that of sexual pleasure. Of course, if we are to hope to influence the sexual culture of young people, it is vital that attention is also focused on the education of young men. Such education should aim to educate young men about the sexual and social needs of young women as well as attempting to redress the balance of responsibility for contraception and sexual health. The young men we interviewed revealed a lack of formal or adequate sex education in general, compared with the young women. It was clear that the peer group had considerable power in constructing their understanding of their masculinity, and that there is a need for their fears of failure and vulnerability to be recognised and licenced (Holland *et al.*, 1993). We identified a potential for greater use of peer education strategies as well as the importance of influencing the messages presented in the media, in particular young women's magazines.

If services and education in sexual health are to be effective they need to incorporate an awareness of the way in which contraceptive choices can influence and structure sexual interaction. This should include an understanding of the ways in which the potential of the pill can reinforce the centrality of spontaneity, and related ideas of loss of control as defining features of sex. The difficulties young women may have in defining sexual encounters as other than steady, despite objective circumstances, also highlights a need to be sensitive to the use of language in contraceptive counselling and education.

Education and services directed at young people must also recognise the problems of consistent long term condom use within 'steady relationships' and the symbolic meanings attributed to condoms. Inevitably this requires the recognition within sexual health education of the limitations of condom use and a willingness to discuss and explain the possibilities of non-penetrative sex to young people in a way which is sensitive to their level of sexual experience. Safer sex strategies which focus exclusively on the use of condoms (a) will have limited effect as we have seen in our discussion of constraints on condom use, and (b) do not offer a long term strategy for young people which is not only positive about sex but which also challenges the disempowering norms of our sexual culture.

Safer sex strategies need to be grounded in a knowledge of both female and male sexuality. The focus on condom use compounds the invisibility of female sexuality in our culture. The lesson from the gay community in terms of safer sex has been that people must feel some ownership of their sexuality before they feel able to control, shape and change their sexual practice. In a sense, it is their marginality in relation to heterosexual culture and the possibilities of procreation which has enabled the redefinition of sexual practice within gay male communities in the light of AIDS. The role of education is central if young heterosexuals are to understand that sexuality and sexual practice are socially constructed and as such can be reconstructed on the basis of self interest and personal growth. An emphasis on what we might call the 'possibilities of non-penetrative sex' is primarily a means by which to encourage young people both individually and collectively to challenge the norms of heterosexual sexual culture rather than a strict alternative to the use of condoms. This is a project with relevance not only for the fight against HIV/AIDS but also for wider issues of effective contraception, informed decision making and sexual health in the broadest sense.

Notes

1 This chapter arises from collective work by the WRAP team (see WRAP team publications in the references). The team are Janet Holland, Caroline Ramazanoglu, Sue Scott, Sue Sharpe and Rachel Thomson. WRAP was funded for two years by the ESRC (1988–1990), and has received additional support from Goldsmiths' College, the Institute of Education Research Fund and the Department of Health. The WRAP team expanded to take in Tim Rhodes when we were funded by the Leverhulme Trust to do a year of research on young men (the Men Risk and AIDS Project, MRAP, 1991–92) using the same methodology as for the study of young women (Holland *et al.*, 1993).
2 Socio-economic class was defined by parental occupations, and overall 47 per cent were middle class and 53 per cent working class, although the proportions varied between the three age groups. 59 per cent of the sample were in education and 41 per cent at work. (Details of the sample are given in Holland, 1993 and Holland *et al.*, 1993).
3 See Sears (1992) for a recent collection of papers on sex education in the USA.
4 A similar relationship between the need to symbolise trust within committed relationships and the non-use of condoms has been documented within gay male relationships (see Weatherburn *et al.*, 1992).
5 See Holland *et al.* (1993) for male strategies to avoid vulnerability in sexual relationships.
6 For a critique and development of the concept of empowerment in the context of gendered power relations see Holland *et al.*, 1992a.

References

ABRAMS, D., ABRAHAM, C., SPEARS, R. and MARKS, D. (1990) 'AIDS invulnerability: Relationships, sexual behaviour and attitudes among 16–19 year olds' in AGGLETON, P., DAVIES, P. and HART, G., *AIDS: Individual, Cultural and Policy Dimensions*, Lewes, Falmer Press.

BURY, J. (1984) *Teenage Pregnancy in Britain*, London, Birth Control Trust.

BURY, J. (1991) 'Teenage sexual behaviour and the impact of AIDS', *Health Education Journal*, **50**(1).

COWARD, R. (1984) *Female Desire: Women's Sexuality Today*, London, Collins/Paladin.

DAY, S., WARD, H. and HARRIS, J. R. W. (1988) 'Prostitute women and public health', *British Medical Journal*, **297**, 1585.

ESTAUGH, V. and WHEATLEY, J. (1990) *Family Planning and Family Well-being*, London, Family Policy Studies Centre.

FARRELL, C. (1978) *My Mother Said . . . the Way Young People Learned About Sex and Birth Control*, London, Routledge and Kegan Paul.

FINE, M. (1988) 'Sexuality, schooling and adolescent females: The missing discourse of desire', *Harvard Educational Review*, **58**(1), 29–53.

FORD, N. (1991) *Regional overview of socio-sexual lifestyles of young people in the south west of England*, Institute of Population Studies, University of Exeter.

FORD, N. (1993) 'The sexual and contraceptive lifestyles of young people: Pt II', *British Journal of Family Planning*, **18**, 119–122.

FORD, N. and BOWIE, C. (1988) 'Sexually related behaviour and AIDS education', *Education and Health*, **Oct.** 86–91.

FORD, N. and MORGAN, K. (1989) 'Heterosexual lifestyles of young people in an English city', *Journal of Population and Social Studies*, **1**(2), January.

GAVEY, N. (1993) 'Technologies and effects of heterosexual coercion' in Wilkinson, S. and Kitzinger, C. (Eds) *Heterosexuality: A 'Feminism and Psychology' Reader*, London, Sage.

General Household Survey (1988) compiled by FOSTER, K., WILMOT, A. and DOBS, J. (OPCS), HMSO.

HOLLAND, J. (1993) *Sexuality and Ethnicity: Variations in Young Women's Sexual Knowledge and Practice*, WRAP Paper 8, London, Tufnell Press.

HOLLAND, J., RAMAZANOGLU, C., SCOTT, S., SHARPE, S. and THOMSON, R. (1990) '"Don't die of ignorance — I nearly died of embarrassment": Condoms in context', WRAP paper 2, London, Tufnell Press.

HOLLAND, J., RAMAZANOGLU, C., SCOTT, S., SHARPE, S. and THOMSON, R. (1992a) 'Pressure, resistance, empowerment: Young women and the negotiation of safer sex', in AGGLETON, P., DAVIES, P. and HART, G., *AIDS: Rights, Risk and Reason*, London, Falmer Press.

HOLLAND, J., RAMAZANOGLU, C., SHARPE, S. and THOMSON, R. (1992b) 'Pleasure, pressure and power: Some contradictions of gendered sexuality', *Sociological Review*, **40**(4), 645–674.

HOLLAND, J., RAMAZANOGLU, C. and SHARPE, S. (1993) *Wimp or Gladiator: Contradictions in Acquiring Masculine Sexuality*, London, Tufnell Press.

HOLLAND, J., RAMAZANOGLU, C., SHARPE, S. and THOMSON, R. (1994) 'Power and desire: The embodiment of female sexuality', *Feminist Review*, **46**, 21–38.

JONES, E. F., *et al.* (1985) 'Teenage pregnancy in developed countries: determinants and policy implications', *Family Planning Perspectives*, **17**(2), 53–63.

LEES, S. (1986) *Losing Out: Sexuality and Adolescent Girls*, London, Hutchinson.

LEES, S. (1993) *Sugar and Spice: Sexuality and Adolescent Girls*, London, Penguin.

NIX, L. M., PASTEUR, A. B., and SERVANCE, M. A. (1988) 'A focus group study of sexually active black male teenagers', *Adolescence*, **23**(91), 741–743.

SCHERING HEALTH CARE (1991) *Sex and Contraception Survey*.

SCHOFIELD, M. (1965) *The Sexual Behaviour of Young People*, London, Longmans.

SEARS, J. T. (Ed.) (1992) *Sexuality and the Curriculum: The Politics and Practices of Sexuality Education*, Columbia University, Teachers College Press.

SPENCER, B. (1984) 'Young men: their attitudes towards sexuality and birth control', *British Journal of Family Planning*, **10**, 13–19.

THOMSON, R. and SCOTT, S. (1991) *Learning About Sex: Young Women and the Social Construction of Sexual Identity*, WRAP paper 4, London, Tufnell Press.

WALDBY, C., KIPPAX, S. and CRAWFORD, J. (1991) 'Equality and eroticism: AIDS and the active/passive distinction', *Social Semiotics*, **1**, 2.

WEATHERBURN, P. *et al.* (1992) *The Sexual Lifestyles of Gay and Bisexual Men in England and Wales*, London, Project Sigma.

WELLINGS, K., FIELD, J., JOHNSON, A.M. and WADSWORTH, J. (1994) *Sexual Behaviour in Britain*, London, Penguin.

WIGHT, D. (1990) 'The impact of AIDS on young people's sexual behaviour in Britain: A literature review', MRC working paper, no. 20, December, 1990.

WILTON, T. and AGGLETON, P. (1991) 'Condoms, coercion and control: Heterosexuality and the limits to HIV/AIDS Education', in AGGLETON, P., HART, G. and DAVIES, P. (Eds) *AIDS: Responses, Interventions and Care*, London, Falmer Press.

Chapter 3

'I'm not Fat, I'm Pregnant': The Impact of Pregnancy on Fat Women's Body Image

Rose Wiles

There is a wide literature that notes that the experience of fatness between the sexes is very different. Research has indicated that women are more likely than men to perceive themselves as fat and to attempt to lose weight (Cox *et al.*, 1987; Gilbert, 1989). One of the explanations for this is the focus on women by the diet and slimming industry (Parham *et al.*, 1986) and the representations of women in the media (Greaves, 1990) in western industrialized societies. Additionally, it has been argued that doctors are more likely to offer advice and treatment to fat women than fat men (Bovey, 1989). There is also evidence that being fat is a far more negative and stigmatized experience for women than it is for men. Fat women have been found to have unpleasant characteristics assigned to them on the basis of their size (Hillier, 1981), to be actively discriminated against in the labour market (Allon, 1980) and to be excluded from full participation in society (Jenkins and Smith, 1987; Greaves, 1990). Such experiences may not be confined to women. However, it is argued that societal disapproval of fatness is aimed chiefly at women rather than men because there is far greater pressure on women to conform to cultural notions of attractiveness. Such notions of attractiveness have, since the 1960s, been closely equated with slimness (Chernin, 1983; Cline and Spender, 1987; Bovey, 1989; Greaves, 1990).

There is anecdotal evidence that the strong social pressure on women to be slim is relaxed to some degree during pregnancy, although there is only a limited amount of research evidence to substantiate this. Clearly pregnancy is a time, perhaps one of the few times during their lives, when it is accepted — and even expected — that women will be fat, at least to some degree. The limited research literature indicates that pregnancy may be a time when fat women could experience their weight in a less negative way due to a greater social acceptability of fatness during pregnancy (Breen, 1981; Orbach, 1984).

While there is little research focusing directly on women's views of their size during pregnancy, research has indicated that the focus on women's physical appearance changes during pregnancy, and that they are viewed differently during this time. Price (1988), for example, notes that there is a shift away from women being viewed as 'seducers' to being viewed as 'producers' during pregnancy. Charles and Kerr (1986) too refer to a move from women's bodies being viewed as 'ornaments' to being viewed as 'functional' during pregnancy. The reduction in the social focus on women's physical appearance during this period may enable fat women to feel less negatively about their size.

However, while pregnancy may be a period when the focus on slimness for women is relaxed socially, there is evidence of a different attitude from the medical profession. Monitoring of weight remains a central feature of ante-natal check-ups even though some clinicians view it as having doubtful value (*General Practitioner*, 1993). Additionally, women of varying sizes are given a considerable amount of advice about diet and 'normal' weight gain during pregnancy. For women who are significantly overweight, advice about diet and weight gain during pregnancy is likely to be even more commonplace. There is a considerable amount of clinical literature noting the health risks for both mother and baby associated with high maternal weight in pregnancy (Abrams and Parker, 1988). Such advice and/or attention from health professionals during pregnancy may negate the more positive feelings that fat women might otherwise have had about their weight resulting from reduced social pressure to be slim.

Research was carried out between 1987 and 1991 to examine fat women's feelings and experiences relating to their weight and their eating practices during and after pregnancy. The word 'fat' was used in this research as this word is viewed as carrying fewer value judgements than words such as 'obese' and 'overweight' which are preferred in clinical literature on the topic (Schoenfielder and Wieser, 1983). The research was designed to discover how women experience being fat and the impact of pregnancy and childbirth on this, focusing on women's subjective feelings and experiences. The research was conducted in two phases: phase one involved interviews with women during late pregnancy, and phase two involved interviews with the same women about six weeks after childbirth. The focus of this chapter is the impact that pregnancy had on the women's feelings about their weight, drawing principally on data collected from the first phase of the research.

Method

The research was designed from a feminist perspective which takes as its starting point the need to be non-hierarchical, non-exploitative and to create a common bond of interest between the researcher and the researched (Stanley and Wise, 1983; Oakley, 1986). Women were interviewed using a semi-structured interview schedule which produced qualitative material. The interviews were carried out in a conversational style with the interviewer making contributions as well as the interviewees. While such a method may not be distinctively feminist it is one that is congruent with feminist principles (Deem, 1986).

A sample of women was identified to take part in the research from the ante-natal records held at a large city hospital and a small rural cottage hospital. Clearly, there are ethical dilemmas in having access to patients' records without their prior knowledge. However, this was the only way that access to this particular group of women could be obtained. A group of community midwives from a health centre in a suburban area identified further potential interviewees from their ante-natal patients, and in the case of these women access to records was not necessary.

The definition of 'fat' used in this study was the attainment of the weight of ninety kilograms by the thirtieth week of pregnancy. This weight has been used in a number of other studies and is viewed as a 'critical' weight when attained in pregnancy and one that is associated with a significant number of medical problems (Gross *et al.*, 1980; Kliegman and Gross, 1985). This definition was chosen both because it is one commonly used in medical literature and because it was felt that women achieving this weight (provided they were not exceptionally tall) would view themselves as 'fat'.

Women obtaining the weight of ninety kilograms or more by the thirtieth week of pregnancy were contacted by post and invited to participate in the study. Enclosed with the letter was a post-card for them to return to indicate whether or not they were willing to participate. In the case of access through the community midwives, the midwives passed on the letters to women fulfilling the ninety kilogram criterion at ante-natal clinics. The letter given to potential interviewees informed them that the research was concerned with the impact of pregnancy on weight and eating and would involve discussing their feelings about their weight and their eating practices before, during and after pregnancy. The women were not told specifically that the research was focused on fat women as it was felt that this might be damaging to their self image. However, they were told clearly what participating in the research would involve and the types of things that would be discussed at the interviews.

The number of women who fulfilled the ninety kilogram criterion was high. In the twelve months spent obtaining a sample, 108 women were identified as potential interviewees. However, the response rate, at thirty-nine per cent, was low probably due to both the sensitive nature of the research and the method of contacting potential interviewees. The women who refused to participate were not followed-up. A comparison of respondents and non-respondents revealed no significant differences between the two groups in terms of age, weight or pregnancy experience. A total of forty-two women agreed to be interviewed and thirty-seven of these were interviewed. The remaining five were unable to be interviewed because they were admitted to hospital before the arranged interview date.

The sample of thirty-seven women interviewed were all white and able-bodied. However, they were not an homogeneous group in terms of age, class, partnership status and number of children. Most of the women (n = 25, 67 per cent) were aged between 21 and 30 years. A further 13 per cent (n = 5) were in the younger age group of between 16 and 20 years; while 19 per cent (n = 7) were in the older age group of between 31 and 35 years. Most (n = 30, 81 per cent) lived with male partners in independent households. Of the rest, six women lived in their parents' home and one woman lived alone. The majority of the women in the study had either no children or only one child (49 per cent, n = 18; and 33 per cent, n = 12 respectively). A smaller number had two (13 per cent, n = 5) or three (5 per cent, n = 2) children. In defining the social class of the sample, the classification devised by Britten and Heath which takes into account both men's and women's employment has been used (see Abbott and Sapsford, 1987). Using this classification, just over half of the sample (54 per cent, n = 20) were class IV. Of the rest eight women (22 per cent) came into class II, five women (13 per cent) came into class I, three women (8 per cent) came into class III and one woman (3 per cent) came into class V.

The women were interviewed in their own homes between the thirtieth and fortieth week of pregnancy. At the interviews, information about the interviewees' backgrounds and past experiences associated with weight and eating were obtained through the use of a life history chart. This chart was divided horizontally into the years of an interviewee's life and vertically into sections covering age, housing, household members, education, occupation, food and eating, and weight and dieting. The aim of using this chart was to get interviewees to talk about their life history in general and in relation to food, eating and weight and this was noted down within the structure of the chart. Following this, a semi-structured questionnaire was used to gather more detailed information about the interviewees' feelings and experiences regarding their weight before and during pregnancy, their experiences of pregnancy in general, and the domestic organization at home. The interviews were tape-recorded and the tapes then transcribed. The data analysis was primarily qualitative.

In relation to the data to be reported in this chapter, the interviewees were asked if they felt satisfied with their weight before pregnancy, and if not, the extent to which they felt their weight affected their views of themselves and their participation in any activities. They were then asked to compare their pre-pregnancy feelings about their weight with their feelings about their weight during pregnancy. Interviewees were asked to state if they felt 'better', 'the same', or 'worse' about their weight during pregnancy than before pregnancy, and were asked in what ways this was so. The interviewees were also asked if the medical professionals with whom they came into contact during pregnancy said anything about their weight, and whether they felt that this had any effect on how they felt about their weight.

Results

Before Pregnancy

The great majority of the interviewees reported a considerable amount of dissatisfaction with their weight before pregnancy. Thirty-one women (84 per cent) reported some dissatisfaction with their weight, and in many cases this dissatisfaction caused them extreme distress. Of the remaining women, only three (8 per cent) were unreservedly satisfied with their weight and a further three (8 per cent) were satisfied as they had dieted and lost weight immediately before becoming pregnant. It was difficult for the women who were dissatisfied with their weight to articulate why they felt that way given that it is a taken-for-granted view held by most people that fat women would prefer to be slim. However, on further discussion, three main areas emerged as presenting difficulties for the women in terms of their weight and were seen as reasons why they would like to lose weight. These areas were not mutually exclusive. The areas were: first, buying and wearing clothes and personal appearance, identified by twenty women; second, taking part in sports and social activities, identified by sixteen women; and, third, comments from family members and others and a desire to lose weight to please them, identified by thirteen women. Surprisingly, no women made reference to health as an area of concern regarding their weight. Thus, even though there has been an increasing emphasis on fatness as an unhealthy state in recent years, these women did not identify this as a primary concern.

The following table shows the numbers of women in each estimated pre-pregnancy weight category who attributed the above three areas as reasons for feeling dissatisfied with their weight.

Table 3.1   Reasons attributed to dissatisfaction with size

	Clothes and personal appearance	Sports and social activities	Comments
70–79 kg (n = 2)	1	1	–
80–89 kg (n = 12)	8	6	4
90–99 kg (n = 11)	8	6	4
100 kg plus (n = 6)	3	3	5
Total	20	16	13

Note: only those women who reported dissatisfaction with their weight are included in this table.

Buying clothes and personal appearance was the most commonly cited reason for wanting to lose weight. This is perhaps not surprising given the focus on women's personal appearance in western industrialized societies. One of the main reasons for this dissatisfaction was that many women felt unable to wear the sorts of clothes that they would have liked to wear. The most prohibitive factor in this appeared to be not the availability of such clothes, but personal sanctioning of them. The sorts of clothes the women felt they would have liked to wear, but felt unable to, were those that reveal expanses of body, such as bikinis, shorts and short skirts. One woman, for example, said: 'I don't dress the way that I want to any more because of my weight. Like, I won't wear shorts or anything like that, no matter how hot it is. Mark says "Oh wear shorts" and I say "no"'.

The act of buying clothes was also cited as a major problem for several reasons. First, fashionable clothes are often not available in larger sizes. Second, clothes in larger sizes are often not available locally or cheaply. Third, the process of actually buying clothes forces women to confront their size in several ways: by having to go to the end of the rack where the large sizes are kept; through having to try clothes on in changing rooms and to view their image in the mirror; and, through the almost inevitable comparisons with other, thinner women who are either shopping for clothes or working as shop assistants. The following comment regarding shopping for clothes was typical:

> Even 'Evans' in town, it's all thin people who work there and they come up to you and say 'can I help you?' and the best thing to say is 'no' because you've got to do it yourself and see how you look with all your lumps and bumps in things. I hate shopping for clothes. I think all fat people do.

In terms of participating in social and sporting activities, 16 of the 31 women who expressed feelings of dissatisfaction about their weight found difficulties in this area to such a degree that their participation was severely restricted or even non-existent. A further eight women felt very self-conscious about their participation but felt able to participate, in many cases, by taking along their children or going with a partner. Sporting activities, and particularly swimming, were viewed as being almost 'out of bounds' for fat women. In most cases the reasons for not participating in such activities seemed to be a view that it was not something that fat people should do, coupled with feelings of self-consciousness, or a fear that someone would draw attention to their weight.

However, it was not only sporting activities from which fat women felt excluded because of their size. Many women reported feeling out of place participating in ordinary social activities such as going to the pub for a drink. Indeed, some women reported that they found going out anywhere led to their feeling out of place and self-conscious. One woman said:

> I don't like going out, to be honest. I really don't like going. Me and my husband rarely go out, you know. I wouldn't dream of going to a disco. But, you know, just going to the pub or anything I'm really conscious of it.

Another woman commented:

> Sometimes when I've been to pubs, I mean, there've been times when I've never taken my coat off, just sat there with my coat on because I've felt so awful. People say 'Why don't you take your

coat off?' and I say 'No, no'. They couldn't think what was wrong.

The third area identified by the women as difficult was that of comments made by partners, family, friends and even strangers regarding their weight. Many of the women noted that they were, or had been, subject to comments from strangers regarding their weight. Such comments served to reinforce fat women's negative views of themselves. Comments from partners, family and friends regarding the women's weight were also fairly common. Thirteen of the thirty-one women who were dissatisfied with their weight received comments regularly and/or wanted to lose weight specifically to please their partners or children. Some comments from partners were particularly hurtful, but, as with the comments from strangers, were seen as justified, as this quotation from one woman illustrates:

> My husband calls me names like 'Jumbo' and things like that . . . He drops hints and that and he says to people 'Oh I only married half of her'. Well it was really, I was only half the size I am now.

It appears, then, that fat women are likely to feel dissatisfied about their weight to some degree. This dissatisfaction stems from their feelings about their attractiveness which is viewed as being greatly diminished because of their size. These feelings are reinforced by the mass media, the diet and slimming industry, and partners, family, friends and even strangers who pass comment on fat women's size. So pervasive is the view that all women must be slim that fat women are likely to accept this view to such an extent that they feel they no longer have a right to respect from others or to fully participate in the social world.

During Pregnancy

While all the women in this study perceived themselves as fat during their pregnancies, the majority reported marked changes in their feelings about their weight during pregnancy from those held prior to pregnancy: fifteen women (41 per cent) reported feeling better about their weight during pregnancy; thirteen women (35 per cent) reported feeling worse; and only nine women (24 per cent) reported not feeling any differently about their weight. The greater social acceptability of fatness during pregnancy emerged as an important factor shaping the women's feelings and this was acknowledged by all the women. For most of the women this meant a liberation from some of the restrictions they placed on their lives before pregnancy. However, while for some women this resulted in their feeling more satisfied with their weight, for others the awareness of the transitory nature of the social acceptability of fatness encouraged them to be wary of allowing themselves to feel their size was more acceptable. For this latter group, the primary factor in determining their feelings was the amount of weight they gained during pregnancy and the effect this weight gain was expected to have on their post-pregnancy weight when fatness would be likely to 're-emerge' as an undesirable state. Comments or advice given by medical professionals also appeared to be a secondary factor.

As the following table shows, all the women reported that their feelings about their weight were affected either by an acknowledgement of the social acceptability of fatness during pregnancy, or by a focus on actual weight gain because of their awareness of the transitory nature of the social acceptability of fatness. Comments or advice by medical professionals were not experienced by all the women, and were reported as a secondary factor which reinforced their feelings about their weight.

Table 3.2 Factors relating to feelings about weight after pregnancy

	Social acceptability of fatness	Focus on weight gain	Medical attitudes
Better (n = 15)	12	3	11
Same (n = 9)	–	9	7
Worse (n = 13)	–	13	11
Total (n = 37)	12	25	29

Acceptance of the social acceptability of fatness
Of the fifteen women who reported feeling better about their weight during pregnancy, 80 per cent (n = 12) reported that they felt this way because they considered it more socially acceptable to be fat during pregnancy. The result of these feelings was that they relaxed some of the constraints on their lives that they experienced before pregnancy. The three main areas that emerged as problematic for the women in terms of their weight before pregnancy declined in importance for these women during pregnancy.

In terms of personal appearance and buying and wearing clothes it was noted that, because fatness is an acceptable part of being pregnant, this was no longer a problematic area of their lives. There are undoubtedly limits on the extent to which fatness is socially acceptable during pregnancy. The social ideal of a pregnant woman's size and shape may not necessarily correspond to the size and shape of the women in this study. Nevertheless, the greater social acceptability of fatness in pregnancy did result in these women feeling far better about their weight in pregnancy than they had before. The result of these feelings was that this group of women felt that the social prohibition of appropriate clothes for fat women was lifted and they felt able to wear clothes, such as shorts and tee-shirts, that they would not wear in a non-pregnant state. Furthermore, buying clothes became a less problematic activity during pregnancy. One woman commented, for example: 'It used to bother me but now, like if I go to the beach, I just put on a big tee-shirt and think 'who cares, I'm pregnant' and people think 'oh that poor pregnant woman'. Another said:

> I feel people can't say 'Oh she's really fat'. People can say 'Oh she's pregnant'. People don't look at you so disgustingly when you're pregnant and wearing something like shorts as they do when you're just vastly overweight.

In addition to the changes in feelings and attitudes relating to their personal appearance, these women also noted that during pregnancy they felt differently about participating in social and sporting activities. Now, some of the women felt able to participate in activities that they had felt excluded from before pregnancy. The most frequently cited activity that the women reported feeling able to participate in during pregnancy was swimming. Interestingly, this was the activity that was most often seen as one to be avoided before pregnancy because of the necessity of having to expose one's size and shape. The following quotation was typical of several women's responses:

> I've only just started going swimming. I find pregnancy a good excuse. I go there deliberately and I think I'm not worried because I'm pregnant. It sounds daft, I don't know if it's in my mind or if people tend to accept me more because I'm pregnant and big, whereas before they'd sort of, well they wouldn't say anything to me, but you get the feeling they're thinking 'look at the size of her'. Now I'm pregnant they probably say 'Doesn't she look wonderful?'.

The third area identified as problematic for the women before pregnancy was that of comments from partners and others and a desire to lose weight to please them. In contrast to the situation before pregnancy, comments from partners, family and friends regarding their weight during pregnancy were few and were not of a critical nature. While several of the women noted that their partners wanted them to lose weight, comments relating to this were generally avoided during pregnancy because this was not seen as a time when anything could be done about it. In addition, where comments were made, these were not taken as seriously by the women as they might have been before pregnancy. Again, the fact that women are expected to be fat during pregnancy probably contributes both to the reduction in the number of comments and the way such comments are received.

Focus on weight gain

The remaining twenty-five women in the study concentrated on their actual weight gain during pregnancy as a focus for their feelings about their weight. All of these women acknowledged the greater social acceptability of fatness during pregnancy but were wary of what they saw as 'falling into the trap' of feeling better about their weight because of this. Like the women in the previous group, these women acknowledged feeling less self-conscious about their dress and personal appearance and feeling more able to participate in social activities. However, this group was aware that the feelings of social acceptability were transitory and would last only for the duration of the pregnancy. Thus, the increased social activity and decreased self-consciousness about their weight did not lead to their feeling better about their weight. These women kept a close eye on the amount of weight they gained during pregnancy and their feelings about themselves were connected to how 'good' or 'bad' they felt their level of weight gain to be. Notions of 'good' and 'bad' levels of weight gain did not correspond solely to medical opinion on acceptable weight gains in pregnancy. Rather, it seemed that personal views of acceptable and unacceptable levels of weight gain were more important. An 'acceptable' level of weight gain was one that was less than the woman envisaged gaining in pregnancy, and one that would enable a woman either to regain her pre-pregnancy weight or to weigh less than she did pre-pregnancy. Conversely, an 'unacceptable' level of weight gain was one that was greater than the woman envisaged, and one that would result in a higher post-pregnancy than pre-pregnancy weight.

Twenty per cent of the women who felt better about their weight ($n = 3$), and all of the women who felt the same about their weight ($n = 9$) as they had done before pregnancy, reported that they did so because their weight gain had been what they perceived as 'good'.

Conversely, all of the women who felt worse about their weight during pregnancy (n = 13) reported that they did so because their weight gain had been what they preceived as 'bad'. One woman, for example, said:

> I suppose you tend to think: oh well, your weight doesn't matter quite so much when you're pregnant. But obviously, at the back of your mind is the fact that you only have nine months of this and that sooner or later you're going to have to pay the price.

Another woman noted:

> I feel like a beached whale at the moment. I feel much worse [than before pregnancy] because I'm so much heavier. I suppose I feel better to a certain extent because it's quite visual that you are pregnant but then I think: my God, you know, will it still be there when I've had the baby and how long will it be there and, you know, will it be really hard to get rid of?

The impact of medical comments and advice

A total of 73 per cent (n = 11) of the women who felt better about their weight during pregnancy, 77 per cent (n = 7) of those who felt the same, and 85 per cent (n = 11) of those who felt worse, reported that comments made, or advice given, about their weight by medical professionals during pregnancy reinforced these feelings. It is necessary here to make a distinction between 'advice' and 'comments'. 'Advice' was defined as medical professionals giving women particular instructions regarding how much weight they should aim to gain or the sort of foods they should eat or avoid eating. 'Comments', on the other hand, were defined as medical professionals making reference to women's weight or diet but not providing instructions as to what they should do about it. Nine women (24 per cent) received comments about their weight from medical professionals. A further twenty women (54 per cent) received advice about their weight from medical professionals: seven of these women sought advice themselves.

Of the nine women who received only comments from medical professionals about their weight during pregnancy, six viewed the comments as derogatory or insulting. The comments appeared to be made quite casually with a lack of awareness of their possible effects. One woman said, for example:

> The midwife said 'You're terribly overweight' and she was really horrible to me. I came out from the clinic crying and my

boyfriend wondered what was wrong. I thought that was a really horrible thing to say to me.

Another woman said: 'I could see what he [her GP] was getting at but it was the way he put it really. He just told me that I was grossly overweight which I didn't agree with really. I was very upset when I came out'.

Seven of the twenty women who received advice, as opposed to comments, regarding their weight and eating during pregnancy sought advice from medical professionals. The remaining thirteen women did not. Being given advice, rather than seeking it, had some impact on the women's feelings about their weight in much the same way that comments did. Again, some women were offended at being given advice because they felt that medical professionals were implying that they were not aware of their weight problem or not trying to do anything about it — a situation which was often far from the truth. One woman was particularly upset by the advice given to her by a hospital consultant:

> He was just downright rude. He said that I should go on a low carbohydrate diet, 'Could you manage that do you think?' he said. And he said that the baby could live off the fat I've got. He just treated me like a complete imbecile and, like, as if I don't look in the mirror and realise that I'm overweight.

Although not all the women responded to advice from medical professionals in this way, of the thirteen women who were given advice, the majority (77 per cent, $n = 10$) reported that medical advice contributed to their feeling the same or worse about their weight than they had done before pregnancy.

Conclusion

The greater social acceptability of fatness during pregnancy was acknowledged and, indeed, generally had a positive impact on body image for most of the women in this study. While not all of the women felt more satisfied with their weight as a result of the greater social acceptability of fatness at this time, such acceptability had an impact on their feelings and attitudes towards their weight during pregnancy, albeit with an awareness by the majority of women that this would be short-lived. This research indicates that pregnancy is a time, perhaps the only time, when fat women's size is approved of because 'being fat' is viewed as a necessary part of being pregnant. Fat women during pregnancy are less likely to feel that they look 'wrong', and one consequence of this is likely to be an easing of self-imposed and societally-imposed restrictions.

The experiences of this group of women appear to be in sharp contrast to the experiences of average-weight women who become pregnant. Research such as that carried out by Oakley (1980) and MacIntyre (1981) has noted that women of average weight express considerable dissatisfaction with their size during pregnancy because of the connotations fatness has with being unattractive (see also Price, 1988). These findings provide further evidence of the importance of body size in women's notion of physical attractiveness, and the importance of physical attractiveness in women's self esteem. It would be interesting to know if congruent findings emerge from research on underweight, or thin, women who become pregnant.

The very negative feelings and experiences of the women in this study before their pregnancies illustrates sharply how notions of physical attractiveness are tied up with notions of acceptability and 'normality' for women in western industrialized societies. Further, it illustrates the extent of distress experienced by women who fall outside such notions of 'normality'.

While many changes have occurred in the position of women over the last forty years or so (at least in the developed world), the emphasis placed on women's physical appearance remains very resistant to change. Indeed, some writers argue that as women have moved increasingly from the private, domestic sphere into public arena, women's sexual attractiveness has become the defining feature of femininity and one that has broadened to include all women rather than just young, single women (Walby, 1990). Certainly, it seems that women are evaluated on the basis of their physical attractiveness by men, other women, and, indeed, themselves, and that much of the sexism and heterosexism they experience is a reflection of this (Measor, 1983; Cunnison, 1989; Walby, 1990). This stress on women's physical appearance can be seen as one of the central pillars of patriarchy in that it defines women as objects whose primary value is in how they look, not who they are or what they can do.

There is no question that a move away from the emphasis on women's physical appearance is crucial for fat women and, indeed, for all women. However, any change is likely to be part of a very long and slow process given that, as Marshment (1993) has argued, images of attractiveness for women are controlled by men, reinforced by the media and the fashion, beauty and slimming industries, and are condoned and accepted by the majority of women.

References

ABBOTT, P. and SAPSFORD, R. (1987) *Women and Social Class*, London, Tavistock.

ABRAMS, B. and PARKER, J. (1988) 'Overweight and pregnancy complications', *International Journal of Obesity*, **12**, 293–303.

ALLON, N. (1980) 'Who is Expert About Fat Discrimination?' Conference paper for The Society For The Study of Social Problems, Philadelphia, USA.

BOVEY, S. (1989) *Being Fat Is Not A Sin*, London, Pandora.

BREEN, D. (1981) *Talking With Mothers*, London, Jill Norman.

CHARLES, N. and KERR, M. (1986) 'Food for feminist thought', *Sociological Review*, **34**, 537–572.

CHERNIN, K. (1983) *The Tyranny of Slenderness*, London, The Women's Press.

CLINE, S. and SPENDER, D. (1987) *Reflecting Men At Twice Their Natural Size*, London, Andre Deutsch.

COX, D. *et al.*, (1987) *The Health and Lifestyles Survey*, London, Health Promotion Research Trust.

CUNNISON, S. (1989) 'Gender joking in the classroom', in ACKER, S. (Ed.) *Teachers, Gender and Careers*, Lewes, Falmer.

DEEM, R. (1986) *All Work and No Play? A Study of Women and Leisure*, Milton Keynes, Open University Press.

General Practitioner (1993) 'Reduce your Antenatal Routine', *General Practitioner*, **1 October**, 1993:31.

GILBERT, S. (1989) *Tomorrow I'll Be Slim: The Psychology of Dieting*, London, Routledge.

GREAVES, M. (1990) *Big and Beautiful: Challenging the Myths and Celebrating Our Size*, London, Grafton.

GROSS, T., SOKOL, R. and KING, K. (1980) 'Obesity in pregnancy: risks and outcome', *Obstetrics and Gynaecology*, **56**, 446–450.

HILLER, D. (1981) 'The salience of overweight in personality characterisation', *Journal of Psychology*, **108**, 233–240.

JENKINS, T. and SMITH, H. (1987) 'Fat liberation', *Spare Rib*, **182**, 14–18.

KLIEGMAN, R. and GROSS, T. (1985) 'Perinatal problems of the obese mother and her infant', *Obstetrics and Gynaecology*, **66**, 299–305.

MACINTYRE, S. (1981) *Expectations and Experiences of First Pregnancy: Report On A Prospective Interview Study of Married Primigravidae In Aberdeen*, Aberdeen, Occasional Paper No. 5, Institute of Medical Sociology.

MARSHMENT, M. (1993) 'The picture is political: representation of women in contemporary popular culture', in RICHARDSON, D. and ROBINSON, V. (Eds) *Introducing Women's Studies*, Basingstoke, Macmillan.

MEASOR, L. (1983) 'Gender and the sciences: pupils' gender-based conceptions of school subjects', in HAMMERSLEY, M., and HARGREAVES, A. (Eds) *Curriculum Practice: Some Sociological Case Studies*, Lewes, Falmer.

OAKLEY, A. (1980) *Women Confined*, Oxford, Martin Robertson.

OAKLEY, A. (1986) *Telling The Truth About Jerusalem*, Oxford, Blackwell.

ORBACH, S. (1984) *Fat Is A Feminist Issue 2*, Feltham, Hamlyn.

PARHAM, E., KING, S., BEDELL, M. and MARTERSTECK, S. (1986) 'Weight control content of women's magazines: bias and accuracy', *International Journal of Obesity*, **10**, 19–27.

PRICE, J. (1988) *Motherhood: What It Does To Your Mind*, London, Pandora.

SCHOENFIELDER, L. and WIESER, B. (1983) *Shadow On A Tightrope: Writings By Women On Fat Oppression*, Iowa, Aunt Lute Books.

STANLEY, L. and WISE, S. (1983) *Breaking Out: Feminist Consciousness and Feminist Research*, London, Routledge and Kegan Paul.

WALBY, S. (1990) *Theorizing Patriarchy*, Oxford, Blackwell.

Chapter 4

Reproductive Health and Reproductive Technology

Pat Spallone

Introduction

The term new reproductive technologies or NRTs covers a whole range of techniques but has come to be associated mostly with *in vitro* fertilisation (IVF) and embryo transfer, where eggs (ova) are removed from women, fertilised in a laboratory dish, and the resulting embryo placed in the woman's womb. The NRTs also include techniques such as GIFT or gamete intrafallopian transfer, where egg(s) and sperm are put in the women's fallopian tube before fertilisation; human embryo research; IVF-assisted surrogacy; genetic screening of embryos; fetal therapy and gene therapy of embryos and fetuses. The term NRTs has also come to include other methods of assisted conception, such as donor insemination (DI) and surrogacy, neither of which is technological nor scientific by definition. DI is the placing of sperm inside the vagina as close to the cervix as possible; it does not require advanced medical knowledge nor technological expertise. Surrogacy is the name given to an arrangement whereby a woman bears a child for another person or couple. Yet, both insemination and surrogacy have been conflated with IVF. They both can, as IVF, be defined medically as infertility treatment; and DI is, as IVF, non-coital reproduction[1].

The aim of this chapter is to consider how scientific priorities help shape the medical development of NRTs, and how those priorities and developments tend to marginalise women's identity as procreators, and women's health needs. When we look at what is actually happening — with infertility and other medical services; in medical research; during medical science conferences and in the ethics debates; or in recent legislation to regulate NRTs — we may notice how questions and priorities often revolve more around what frontier science and new technology can do (never asking why it should be doing it like this); and their effects on an abstract concept of the family and society.

IVF is the main focus of my attention because it defined the 'newness' of the NRTs technologically and socially. Removing women's eggs was the precondition for developments such as human embryo research. Furthermore, IVF changed the possibilities and our conception of what is normal. For example, now that eggs can be removed from women the question arises, 'Who is the biological mother, the woman who bears a child or the woman from whom the egg came?'. These are social experiments of unprecedented proportions.

Also, the social controversy over IVF prompted the British Government to charge a Committee of Inquiry on Human Fertilisation and Embryology in 1982 to investigate IVF and human embryo research, surrogacy and insemination. The Report of this Committee, the famous Warnock Report (1984) chaired by philosopher Mary Warnock, was the basis of recent legislation, the Human Fertilisation and Embryology Act 1990, and the earlier Surrogacy Arrangements Act 1985, which banned commercial surrogacy arrangements.

In focusing on IVF, I am not so much concerned with what the technology can do, but how scientifically-defined priorities affect health developments, the professional assessment of the usefulness and safety of NRTs, and the social reverberations of the NRTs and assisted reproduction. Scientific priorities help shape attitudes, ethical concerns, and real services. I am interested in the interplay of ethics, research developments, and clinical services; and how scientific priorities compare and contrast with some feminist concerns. My discussion is organised as follows:

- The ethics: and how the ethics debate affects developments, and the perception and representation of clinical and social problems.
- Developments in the clinic: the logic of risk.
- Medical services: infertility services as an example.

The Ethics of NRTs

The Embryo as Human Subject

The dominating ethical concern in the social debate over IVF has been the human status of the human embryo. It is an old preoccupation in Western intellectual tradition, dating at least from the time of the ancient Greeks who pondered the question, 'When does human life begin?' Greek philosophers and physicians imagined states of non-being and being in embryonic development (although they had no concept of embryology as we know it). Aristotle decided that male embryos 'form' or become 'being' at forty days gestation; while females, imperfect males, 'form' at eighty days. The notion that life begins at some moment in development became part of Western thought and the basis for legal sanctions imposed against abortion.

In the IVF debate, that preoccupation with the embryo is posed as the question, 'How far should society allow science to go experimenting with embryos and handling them?' An editorial in the magazine *New Scientist* declared, 'The important ethical question is: should scientists conduct research on live human embryos? When do embryos become people?' (*New Scientist*, 1982, p. 290).

By contrast, women have not been explicitly identified as a central subject of IVF despite the fact that embryology, after all, is the study of pregnancy (a uniquely female experience). There has been little recognition of women's bodies in the conceptualisation of NRTs. One argument which kept cropping up in early scientific rhetoric is that removing women's eggs is the same as acquiring men's sperm, so there is no ethical dilemma in fact. An editorial defending the cause of embryo research in the international science journal *Nature* stated:

> Uneasiness that the ova are obtained artificially by a relatively simple procedure is understandable but indefensibly irrational, given the widespread and apparently acceptable practice of artificial insemination with husband's sperm. (*Nature*, 1982, p. 475)

Firstly, this argument ignores the obviously different processes involved in procuring eggs and sperm: the hormone and drug regimes for ovarian stimulation, surgical egg removal, the months and even years of a woman's physical and emotional commitment to IVF treatment which affects everything else. These are not seen as issues. To suggest that these processes mean something is seen as 'indefensibly irrational'.

Secondly, the *Nature* editorial's argument ignores the revolutionary social and cultural implications of removing women's eggs and embryos from the female body, namely, the question of biological motherhood, 'Who is the mother?'. Notice too how the *Nature* editorial's conceptualisation of the problem favours a male experience of reproduction where the reproductive cell (sperm, egg) is destined to be separated from the body.

The logic of the *Nature* editorial is one example of how the implications for women have not been seen as a main issue of IVF ethics. Rather, repeatedly, the ethical questions in reproductive medicine tend to be about state-of-the-art techniques (such as egg removal), and questions which arise such as who owns the embryo?, is it a person?, and should doctors be allowed to use babies without brains for organ transplants? (Spallone, 1988). These are all relevant questions, but they should not be allowed to take priority over questions regarding medical, emotional and social welfare of women (and children, and men involved), and women's status as the primary human subject of NRTs.

For instance, emotional commitment to IVF and other infertility programmes is part of the reality of treatment, as anyone working on programmes and as the women involved may point out. It can be difficult for some women and couples to make the decision to stop trying after repeated failures at getting pregnant.

Social Implications of Embryo Protection

Certain of the social implications of embryo-centred ethics became clear in the context of the Embryology Bill 1989 (now an Act). The Embryology Bill is meant in part to be protectionist legislation, but it was mostly concerned with protection of embryos, not women.

The most publicised clauses in the bill concerned whether or not human embryo research should be allowed. Human embryo research is experimentation on, or observation of, IVF embryos, the result of fertilisation of egg and sperm outside the woman's body. MPs had a choice between two clauses. They could vote either for allowing regulated embryo research up until fourteen days after fertilisation, or against human embryo research altogether. These were the only options available, grounded in terms of embryo protection. They voted for allowing regulated embryo research (Spallone, 1990).

There were several Parliamentary attempts to use the revealingly dubbed 'Embryo Bill' to lower the time of legal abortion despite the fact that Mary Warnock called these attempts 'evil', and tried to distance the two subjects, abortion and embryo research (Warnock, 1991). Abortion and embryo research will never be separated in an embryo-centred world. Indeed, the scientific view of IVF is embryo-centred,[2] and in conjunction with the Embryology Bill, Parliament lowered the legal upper time limit of abortion from twenty-eight days as it previously stood to twenty-four days. (A twenty-four day limit had been supported by medical authorities in Britain for years, independently of the debate on NRTs. Still, the legal change significantly was made in the context of the Embryology Bill.)

The implications of an Embryology Act founded on implicit notions of embryo protection is open for interpretation. I often point to the United States, where women have been forced to have Caesarean section births against their wills by doctors who have procured court orders on the basis of their professional judgement that the fetus, at twenty-four weeks or older, would otherwise be endangered. The legal basis for such treatment of women, which peaked in the 1980s (see Spallone, 1989), came from legal interpretations of the US Supreme Court's ruling of *Roe* v *Wade*. Fetal protection was never written directly into US law, but was inferred from the *Roe* v *Wade* decision whose main effect was to liberalise abortion in the USA. Although the same situation is not likely in the UK, the example shows how embryology legislation may endanger women's rights.

My general point is that from the beginning of the ethics debate on NRTs, women were marginalised as the primary human subject of NRTs, as the human being whose physical presence is the prerequisite of IVF, human embryo research, fetal therapies, gene therapy of embryos, genetic screening of embryos, expansion of prenatal screening tests, and so on.[3]

A Second Social Implication of the NRTs: The Fit Parent

The ethics of the embryo is linked with the ethics of the family, and socially as well as clinically women have been subordinated to some extent. Consistently, many IVF advocates, including the science journal *Nature*, emphasised throughout the ethical debates of the early 1980s that IVF was for wives, and emphasised the particular social context in which conception and pregnancy would be enabled.

The Warnock Report made this concern with the stability of the heterosexual nuclear family explicit. It asserted that all forms of assisted conception with which it was concerned — IVF and donor insemination — were for heterosexual couples living together in a stable relationship, married or not. Donor insemination is now controlled by the same medical and government authorities as for IVF, not because insemination requires scientific expertise as does IVF; not because it carries the medical risks that IVF interventions do; not because it is open to commercial exploitation as is surrogacy; but, we must conclude, because of anxiety over the free use of insemination, for example by women using it as a reproductive option.

During Parliamentary debates over the Embryology Bill, insemination became the subject of vituperative comments on lesbian sexuality, although attempts to create discriminatory clauses in the bill failed. Meanwhile, *broad* questions of health care and priorities in reproductive medicine were not part of the Warnock Inquiry's remit, nor part of the medical science debate on the NRTs, nor part of the parliamentary debate on the Embryology Bill. In fact, neither were *narrow* questions of health care part of these debates, questions such as the clinical risks for women of the new techniques, as well as the not-so-new medical approaches used in conjunction with IVF.

Developments in the Clinic: The Logic of Risk

As with any medical intervention of the calibre of IVF, immediate and long-term risks are of concern. The most publicised effect of IVF in Britain has been the high incidence of triplets, quadruplets, quintuplets or more — higher order multiple birth children. The risk of multiple pregnancy is increased by the practice of ovulation stimulation in infertility treatment, and more recently with the IVF practice of inserting multiple embryos — two or more embryos — into a woman's womb. The reason for inserting more than one embryo is to increase the chances of pregnancy occurring. When a single embryo is inserted, there is a much lower chance of becoming pregnant. The need for a better understanding of the entire situation became apparent from 1986 onwards as 'neonatal paediatricians voiced their concern about the incidence, risks and consequences of multiple births and their effects on neonatal services' (Price, 1991, p. 8). Those concerns became the subject of a national study whose findings are now available to clinicians faced with decisions relating to the medical management of infertility (Botting *et al.*, 1990; see also Price 1992a, 1992b).

A second category of risk, though less immediately evident or certain as multiple birth, is short- and long-term risks from taking fertility drugs and hormones routinely used in IVF. I will discuss these further because I believe that they provide an important example of how easily the risk of a drug can be dismissed either as irrelevant or as a technical factor which medical science can deal with, when neither medicine nor science is dealing with it very well. I do not wish to overinflate such risks, but to consider the way in which these sorts of risks have been treated in the debate on NRTs.

How Much Risk is Too Much Risk?

Combinations of ovarian stimulation drugs are administered to stimulate and control the woman's menstrual cycle for IVF. Super-ovulation is the process by which the woman's ovaries produce many eggs per cycle, instead of the usual one egg. At first, four, six or eight ova were being extracted from a woman's ovaries. Then came reports of fourteen, then up to forty-one and sixty-one ova removed from a woman's ovaries at one 'superovulated' cycle (Simons, 1991).

The medical literature has chronicled cases of women who suffer ill effects of the fertility drug regimens, sometimes grave effects, including depression, cancer, high rates of miscarriage, ovarian cysts, damage to the ovaries and menstrual cycle, hyperstimulation of the ovaries, possible ovarian cancer. (Ashkenazi *et al.*, 1987; Börlum and Maigaard, 1989; Carter and Joyce, 1987; Fishel and Jackson, 1989; Kaaja *et al.*, 1989; Kulkarni and McGarry, 1989; St Clair Stephenson, 1991; Wagner and St Clair Stephenson, 1989; see also Klein and Rowland, 1988; Klein, 1989.)

Although, for example, the correlation of ovarian cancer and fertility drugs is not proved beyond a shadow of a doubt, there is medical cause to believe that it may be a factor (Carter and Joyce, 1987). These cases are thought to be very rare, and adverse effects such as hyperstimulation are controllable, but the point is that such risks have not been adequately recognised as part of the social and clinical assessment of NRTs.

Fertility drugs have been administered for infertility treatment well before IVF, and IVF practitioners were aware of certain risks. Test-tube baby pioneer Robert Edwards noted back in 1974, four years before the first IVF birth, that 'the two serious risks [from gonadotrophins or clomiphene used for ovarian stimulation] were known to be hyper-stimulation of the ovary and multiple births' (Edwards, 1974, p. 6).

At the Second International Conference on Philosophical Ethics in Reproductive Medicine (PERM II) in 1991 at the University of Leeds, I voiced my concerns over the lack of recognition of these risks as a medical ethics issue when assessing the worth of expanding the applications of NRTs. I made the plea during discussion time after the first speaker, Professor Peter Braude, Senior Lecturer in Obstetrics and Gynaecology in Cambridge, spoke on embryo therapy, 'What Can Be Done?'. He argued the worth of embryo therapy in terms of the status of the embryo alone. His reply to me was that the ethics of using fertility drugs was 'irrelevant' (his word) to PERM's concerns. No one challenged his position. Yet later that same day at that same conference another speaker used the well-known and sometimes life-threatening risk of ovarian hyperstimulation syndrome to argue a case for freezing IVF embryos (freezing human embryos raised ethical concerns when the capability was realised).

Dr Eric Simons of Cromwell IVF and Fertility Centre, in his presentation of 'Ethical Consideration of Embryo Freezing During Augmented Fertility Treatment', explained that hyperstimulation of a woman's ovaries was a known risk in IVF. Hence, he argued, using frozen embryos for embryo transfer at a later date, during a woman's unstimulated cycle, was a better IVF option; a risk factor which might interfere with a successful outcome would thus be removed. In his logic, the risk of ovarian hyperstimulation syndrome suggested to him another permutation of IVF, but not a reassessment of the drug regimens themselves. For him, the known risk was deemed appropriate to an ethics discussion, and its recognition led him to a favourable conclusion regarding the expansion of NRTs. In this case, a known risk of ovarian stimulation is relevant; in another case, it is irrelevant. My concern remains: is it actually a good idea to create a line of therapy — embryo therapy — which demands that more women contemplate IVF reproduction, with all of its attendant problems? Why are known and even unknown adverse effects and complications not consistently part of the IVF discussion?

The DES Story and IVF

If this were the first time in history we were faced with the difficulty of making judgements about how much risk is too much risk, then perhaps I would understand the lack of critical attention. But it isn't the first time. Consider DES (diethylstilbestrol), which was once prescribed to women as an anti-miscarriage drug during pregnancy. It was rushed into use with little evidence of efficacy and safety in the late 1950s. It was marketed as a kind of pregnancy vitamin pill that could make 'healthy pregnancies healthier'.

It took some twenty years to pinpoint that DES is linked to a higher risk of a rare form of vaginal cancer in daughters of women who took it, fertility problems in their daughters and sons, and breast cancer in the women themselves, among other adverse effects. The link was made only because the form of cancer found in the daughters was so rare. There could be little doubt about the immediate cause.

Daughters of women who were prescribed DES during pregnancy may be found on infertility programmes seeking treatments. One of the DES-related non-cancerous abnormalities which can make it difficult to carry a pregnancy to full term is a condition called 'T-shaped uterus' where there is reduced elasticity, and which is seen in some DES daughters (Laitman, 1990).

The risks of cancer and infertility for DES daughters goes particularly unrecognised in this country, emphasises Michelle Cowen of the DES Action group in Britain:

> We have to get our information from Canada or the United States. Some individual doctors are sympathetic when a DES daughter becomes known, but we believe there are a lot more women at risk than the Department of Health estimates, and they fail to take on board the necessity of regular and careful screening for women at risk ... Women aren't told about the possible risk of infertility from DES. If DES daughters knew, they could be prepared if they find they are having difficulty getting pregnant. (Cowen, 1994)

Considering that the medical literature contains at least some warning of adverse effects of certain fertility drugs, and considering the DES lesson, why then are not the risks taken on board in the debate on NRTs? For one, hyperstimulation syndrome can be avoided by careful monitoring, and some practitioners argue that the best clinics will always avoid the risk. In addition, many if not most IVF doctors and scientists argue that data does not support the claim of risk, although others suggest that risks should be taken more seriously. (See Bromwich and Walker, 1989; Dalton and Lilford, 1989; Edwards *et al.*, 1989; for counter-replies to medical claims of risks.)

A co-founder of DES Action International, and a DES daughter herself, Anita Direcks has written about the connections she sees between DES and IVF:

> One of the most important concerns I have in regard to IVF is about the long-term effects for mother and child: the consequences of the hormonal treatment, the medium [the liquid solution of nutrients in which the egg and sperm are placed] and so on ... We should question each step in the IVF procedure ... Inadequate information is given about the experimental character of the medical intervention ... causes of fertility problems are ignored ... Both technologies, DES and

IVF, did not have to be proven safe for women. The idea is that it is safe until it is proven otherwise. (Direcks, 1987, pp. 163–164)

Another Risk: The Hepatitis Outbreak

Soon after Direcks said this, a case which illustrates her concern occurred — an outbreak of hepatitis among 172 women in the IVF programme at a hospital in The Netherlands. The culture medium which was used to grow eggs and embryos became contaminated with hepatitis B virus. The source of the virus was the human blood serum which was added to the growing medium. Adding human blood serum has been a common practice in IVF, but there is no scientific evidence which warrants including blood serum in the media; it was just thought to provide a protein source or some other factor which might help fertilisation and maintenance of the embryo.

Medical ethicist Helen Bequart Holmes observed the case and commented that the ultimate cause of the incident was not just sloppiness and carelessness in the Dutch IVF laboratory but the 'experimental nature of IVF, the hey, what-shall-we-try-next, hocus-pocus, and the gambling, risk-taking behaviour that it tends to foster, which allows well-trained scientists around the world to carry out cavalier trial-and-error experiments' (Holmes, 1989, p. 36).

The example illustrates the way in which women, although perhaps implicitly recognised as clinical subjects of IVF from the beginning, are not adequately identified or protected as such subjects (rather, the embryo is, or apparently is).

Nothing is perfect. Every medical intervention carries some risk. But an easy acceptance that 'nothing is perfect' can too easily reduce problems to simple human imperfection, making it difficult to address questions of medical accountability and social forces (such as overarching scientific priorities) which help shape treatments.

Services

This brings me to the question of how NRTs fit into existing medical services and affect them. I will take infertility services as my main example to illustrate our need for a context-sensitive policy, as well as a better concept of medical success.

Infertility was the first medical indication or application for IVF, the assumption being that it is by definition progress in infertility treatment.[4] But if we actually look at infertility services, this assumption is not borne out. In a report on infertility services for the Greater London Association of Community Health Councils, Naomi Pfeffer and Allison Quick noted:

> We gained a strong impression that, since the publication of the Warnock Report, the quality of treatment that the majority of the infertile men and women receive within the NHS has deteriorated in some areas although, or even because, *in vitro* fertilisation and embryo transfer have been introduced (Pfeffer and Quick, 1988, p. 12).

Pfeffer and Quick concluded that recent growth of infertility services has been the haphazard result of individual consultant's interests, but that systematic organisation of services is lacking.

Consider how infertility was defined from the outset as a biological malfunction. The Warnock Report asserted:

> an inability to have children is a malfunction . . . In addition, the psychological distress that may be caused by infertility in those who want children may precipitate a mental disorder warranting treatment. It is, in our view, *better to treat the primary cause* of such distress than to alleviate the symptoms (Warnock Report, 1984, p. 9, my emphasis).

By the primary cause they mean the biological malfunction. But the biological malfunction is not the primary cause of infertility. Medically speaking, the primary causes of infertility are many and varied, for example, in many women pelvic infections not caught in time. In fact, research and services are necessary at precisely this level; the additional bonus of attention to cause, prevention and primary health care is that it does not bring the complex ethical dilemmas, social control dilemmas and cultural dilemmas and uncertainties of the NRT route.

Furthermore, a problem with the disease model — the malfunctioning parts model — is that psychological and social aspects of involuntary childlessness are relegated to a subsidiary role. Or, the psychological and social aspects end up becoming evidence to support the use of more NRTs, rather than becoming a reason to address the psychological and social factors themselves. For example:

a. there are often factors at play for an individual which pre-date her (or his) infertility, factors with which that person may require help;

b. having a baby by assisted conception does not alleviate all of the distress of infertility (IVF doesn't cure or reverse infertility, and the person may still be distressed by their inability to reproduce);

c. the purely technological approach has left little or no room for women in the programmes, or men for that matter, to acknowledge ambiguous feelings over parenthood or over the treatment itself.

Recognition of these and other factors at the level of services can mean looking at the way informed consent is treated when an individual is caught up in the success syndrome where success is measured by getting a baby at the end of the line. If success means something more, if it means working through and thriving, the picture would look different.

Taking the scientific end of infertility treatment as one distinct category, uninformed by wider interpersonal and social dimensions, diminishes the possibilities. The NRTs (as they have been allowed to be developed) have narrowed the definition of cause and prevention. The 'biological malfunction' becomes the cause of people's distress; IVF and related methods thus become the solution.

It is worth thinking about how a similar logic is occurring in the use of genetic interventions in reproduction, such as expansion of genetic screening tests, or the new gene therapies (gene therapy may be defined as genetic engineering of human cells when treating a medical condition). Genes become identified as a cause of more health problems, and so genetic technology becomes the solution (Spallone, 1992). Genetic screening of IVF embryos is generally well accepted in the medical science world; and while the UK Government's Clothier Report on the Ethics of Gene Therapy recommended a ban on genetic engineering in embryos at this time, they also suggested that genetic risk warrants the idea of embryo gene therapy. We are left with more reasons for women to contemplate IVF pregnancy. All of the (undiscussed) questions of NRTs remain and more, such as: is the expansion of genetic cause and genetic solutions in medicine marginalising other causes of, and solutions to, disabilities and illnesses?; is antenatal screening itself adequately delivered and with regard to its widest social aspects?; how do we as a society view disability, and the relationship of reproduction to it?

Some Final Words

The social and biological reverberations of NRTs are extraordinary, but not entirely the way that a wholly scientific viewpoint sees the problems and promises. In many respects, the NRTs are not all that new, and are prone to continue a problem which feminist writers on reproductive medicine have located before. In the words of social scientist Barbara Katz Rothman, 'There's this incredible lack of faith in the body. We start feeling that we all need *in vitro* fertilisation and Caesarean sections to get babies in and out' (cited in Hopkins, 1985).

It is unsatisfactory to take each new development as a neutral technique which can be added or not to the repertoire of medical services. Rather, we need to put back the context, and reframe central questions. Instead of asking, 'How can NRTs be used in society?', we need to ask, 'How best can health concerns of fertility and infertility, genetic and congenital illnesses, and disability, be addressed? How best can medical science contribute?'

In this chapter, I have explored certain avenues of thought on the NRTs, reaching back to debates and developments of the past decade. As I finalised it for publication, months after it was first given as a talk, a good many controversial NRT developments have gained public attention: should parents be allowed to choose the sex or race of their children?; should eggs from human fetuses be used in IVF?; should 'older' women after menopause be allowed to have IVF? The level of public discussion remains all too familiar: centred on state-of-the-art technical capabilities; morally preoccupied with the definition of the life of the fetus; with the ubiquitous voices of medical science spokespersons instructing through the media that we should not be afraid of progress. The clinical services themselves remain largely in the private sector, and although a formal regulatory mechanism is in place (the aptly named Human Fertilisation and Embryology Authority), and although government committees are set up to investigate certain developments, they all appear locked into a mind-set which accepts the claims and terms of scientific progress as played out in the political arena. Certainly, in my experience, they do not take on board the concerns put before them by groups with which I have been involved. Where are the questions about, say, the uses of medical science in social engineering? When one raises such questions in the most authoritative formal meetings and conferences which are meant to be a forum for debate, the incomprehension is palpable. 'It's like taking your clothes off in public', someone once said to me.

Reframing questions and placing wider concerns on the agenda is a tall order, but not impossible. It continues to impress on me during casual discussions or in meetings of smaller groups, that so many people actually are worried and concerned about these wider issues. Practically and immediately we have to wonder about the silences and the difficulties of having a deep and relevant public debate on these matters, which presupposes working through these areas for ourselves as well.

Notes

1   All of the terms given are complex and imperfect. The term new reproductive technologies 'can be confusing and somewhat misleading' (McNeil, 1993, p. 483). In its place, other phrases — such as assisted conception, assisted reproduction, assisted procreation, and procreative technologies — are often used and may be more appropriate. However, for the purposes of this article in which I am particularly interested in exploring developments in reproductive medical science, the term NRTs is the most suitable, I think. It reflects the way in which scientific expertise and knowledge dominates the social parameters of female fertility. Maureen McNeil recognises another reason for using the label NRTs: 'recent developments in this field suggest that a desire for *'reproduction'* (however unrealizable) might fuel some forms of involvement with this technology, particularly amongst some male scientists and doctors' (McNeil, 1993, p. 484).

      Similarly with other terms: recently I have seen the term assisted insemination (AI) used rather than donor insemination. Rather than 'surrogacy', the Canadian Royal Commission on New Reproductive Technologies used 'preconception agreement . . . where a woman agrees to conceive and carry a pregnancy in order to hand over the child to a commissioning person to raise' (Canadian Royal Commission, 1993, p. 14).

2   From my researches in this area, I would argue that the scientific community had no choice but to be embryo-centred. The moral debate became centred on the embryo. If scientific advocates of NRTs rejected the terms of the debate, they would either appear to be amoral Frankensteins, or they would be left with having to recognise women as a central human subject of embryology, which complicates things even further. The architecture and psychology of the debate — with its embryo/progress polarity and its marginal representation of women — is complicated, but it largely remains oriented on what science knows about embryos. Science informs society about the status of the embryo. On the other hand, science cannot claim such a superior all-embracing knowledge of the status of women.

3   Sarah Franklin's work illuminates that the problem is the selective representation of women's needs, desires and feelings. Women's voices are heard in the debate on IVF, but 'they are particular voices, to the exclusion of others'. Certain women's voices are excluded and certain representations of women's experience are excluded. A reason to be 'somewhat sceptical is that the exaltation of certain reproductive needs is dramatically at odds with the actual state of reproductive health care facilities for women in Britain' (Franklin, 1992).

4   See Pfeffer, 1993, for a history of infertility treatment and its medical research over the century.

DES Action in Britain may be contacted through Women's Health, 52 Featherstone St, London EC1. Tel: 071 251 6580.

References

((C) designates correspondence to journal editors)

ASHKENAZI, J., FELDBERG, D., BENDAVID, M., SHELEF, M., DICKER, D. and
GOLDMAN, J.A. (1987) 'Ovum pickup for *in vitro* fertilisation: A case of
mechanical infertility?', *Journal of In Vitro Fertilisation and Embryo Transfer*,
4, 242–5.

BÖRLUM, K.-B. and MAIGAARD, S. (1989) (1 July), 'Transvaginal oocyte aspiration and
pelvic infection', *The Lancet*, 53.

BOTTING, B.J., MACFARLANE, A.J. and PRICE, F.V. (1990) *Three, Four or More: A
Study of Triplets and Higher Order Births*, London, HMSO.

BROMWICH, P. and WALKER, A. (C), (1989, 2 December), *The Lancet*, 1327.

CANADIAN ROYAL COMMISSION ON NEW REPRODUCTIVE TECHNOLOGIES (1993)
December, Update. (P.O. Box 1566, Station B, Ottowa, Canada K1P 5R5; for
*Proceed with Care: The Final Report of the Royal Commission On New
Reproductive Technologies*, 1993, contact Canada Communications Group
Publishing, Ottawa, Ontario, K1A 0S9).

CARTER, M.E. and JOYCE, D.N. (1987) 'Ovarian carcinoma in a patient hyper-
stimulated by gonadotrophin therapy for *in vitro* fertilisation: A case report',
Journal of In Vitro Fertilisation and Embryo Transfer, 4(2), 126–128.

Committee of Inquiry into Human Fertilisation and Embryology, Report, (1984)
London, HMSO. Reprinted in WARNOCK, M. (1985) *A Question of Life*,
London, Basil Blackwell.

Committee on The Ethics of Gene Therapy, Report (1992) Cm 1788, London, HMSO.

COWEN, M. (1994) personal communication, 17 January.

DALTON, M. and LILFORD, R.J. (C) (1989, 2 December), *The Lancet*, 1327.

DIRECKS, A. (1987) 'Has the lesson been learned? The DES story and IVF', in
SPALLONE, P. and STEINBERG, D.L. (Eds) *Made to Order: The Myth of
Reproductive and Genetic Progress*, Oxford, Pergamon.

EDWARDS, R.G. (1974) 'Fertilisation of human eggs *in vitro*: morals, ethics and the
law', *Quarterly Review of Biology*, 49, 3–26.

EDWARDS, *et al.* (C) (1989, 2 December), *The Lancet*, 1328.

FISHEL, S. and JACKSON, P. (1989) 'Follicular stimulation for high tech pregnancies:
are we playing it safe?', *British Medical Journal*, 299, 309–311.

FRANKLIN, S. (1992) 'Contested Conceptions: A Cultural Account of Assisted
Reproduction', PhD thesis, Faculty of Arts, University of Birmingham.

HOLMES, H.B. (1989) 'Hepatitis — Yet another risk of *in vitro* fertilisation?',
*Reproductive and Genetic Engineering: Journal of International Feminist
Analysis*, 2(1) 29–37.

HOPKINS, E. (1985, 11 August), 'High Tech Pregnancies', *The Newsday Magazine*,
reprinted with permission in *Midwives Information and Resource Service
Information Pack* (1986) No. 1.

HUMAN FERTILISATION AND EMBRYOLOGY BILL (1989), London, HMSO.

KAAJA, R., SIEBERG, R., TIITINEN, A. and KOSKIMIES, A. (1989) 'Severe ovarian
hyperstimulation syndrome and deep venous thrombosis', *The Lancet* (28
October), 1043.

KLEIN, R. (Ed.) (1989) *Infertility: Women Speak Out About Their Experiences*,
London, Pandora.

KLEIN, R. and ROWLAND, R. (1988) 'Women as test-sites for fertility drugs:
Clomiphene citrate and hormonal cocktails', *Reproductive and Genetic
Engineering: Journal of International Feminist Analysis*, 1(3), 251–274.

Pat Spallone

KULKARNI, R. and MCGARRY, J. M. (1989) Follicular stimulation and ovarian cancer, *British Medical Journal*, **299**, 740.

LAITMAN, C. (1990) 'DES on Prescription: It's Time for Europe to Act', *Scientific European*, (October) 27–29.

MCNEIL, M. (1993) 'New Reproductive Technologies: Dreams and Broken Promises', *Science as Culture*, 3(17), 483–506.

Nature, (1982) 'The future of the test tube baby', **299**, 475–476.

New Scientist, (1982, 4 February) 'Test-tube baby under microscope', 290.

Pfeffer, N. and Quick, A. (1988) *Infertility Services: A Desperate Case*, a report for the Greater London Association of Community Health Councils, 100 Park Village East, London NW1 3SR.

Pfeffer, N. (1993) *The Stork and the Syringe: A Political History of Reproductive Medicine*, London, Polity.

PRICE, F. (1991) 'Clinical Practice and Clinical Concern', presented at the seminar: *Kinship and the New Reproductive Technologies: Anthropological Perspectives on Assisted Kinship*, University of Manchester, 19 September 1991. [See Price, F. (1993) 'Beyond expectation: clinical practices and clinical concerns', in EDWARDS, J., FRANKLIN, S., HIRSCH, E., PRICE, F. and STRATHERN, M. (Eds) *Technologies of Procreation: Kinship in the Age of Assisted Conception*, Manchester and New York, Manchester University Press.]

PRICE, F. (1992a) 'Having Triplets, Quads or Quints: Who Bears the Responsibility?', in STACEY, M. (Ed.) *Changing Human Reproduction*, London, Sage.

PRICE, F. (1992b) '"Isn't She Coping Well?": Providing For Mothers of Triplets, Quadruplets and Quintuplets', in ROBERTS, H. (Ed.) *Women's Health Matters*, London, Routledge.

ST CLAIR STEPHENSON, P. (1991) 'The Risks Associated with Ovulation Induction', *Iatrogenics*, **1**, 7–16.

SIMONS, E. G. (1991) 'Ethical Consideration of Embryo Freezing During Augmented Fertility Treatment', a talk presented 15 April, The Second International Conference on Philosophical Ethics in Reproductive Medicine, University of Leeds, 14–19 April 1991.

SPALLONE, P. (1988) 'Report on the First International Conference on Philosophical Ethics in Reproductive Medicine', 18–22 April 1988. *Reproductive and Genetic Engineering*, **1**(3), 309–312.

SPALLONE, P. (1989) *Beyond Conception: The New Politics of Reproduction*, London, Macmillan; Massachusetts, Bergin & Garvey.

SPALLONE, P. (1990) 'Of eggs and men', *Trouble and Strife*, **18**, 15–19.

SPALLONE, P. (1992) *Generation Games: Genetic Engineering and the Future for Our Lives*, London, The Women's Press; Philadelphia, Temple University Press.

WAGNER, M. and ST CLAIR STEPHENSON, P. (1989, 28 October) 'Are *In Vitro* Fertilization and Embryo Transfer of Benefit to All?', *The Lancet*, 1027–1329.

WARNOCK, M. (1991, 29 October), 'Why abortion clause in embryo bill is "evil",' London, *The Observer*.

[Warnock Report (1984), see *Committee of Inquiry...*].

Chapter 5

Waged Work and Well-being

Lesley Doyal

One of the most striking developments of the post-war period has been the increase in female work outside the home. Though women still carry the major burden of domestic labour worldwide, they also make up over one third of the paid labour force (United Nations, 1991, pp. 88–96). For most women, staying at home is no longer an option, and many move in and out of employment as financial need, personal preference, domestic circumstances and job opportunities dictate. Since their place in the labour force is now well established, we need to assess the implications this has for women's health.

For decades, middle-class married women in the developed countries were threatened with sterility, cancer, madness and all manner of other diseases if they left their homes for the world of work (Ehrenreich and English, 1979). However, it was not until the 1970s that scientific investigation into the health effects of women's employment was undertaken on any scale (Chavkin, 1984; Frankenhaueser *et al.*, 1991; Nathanson, 1975; Repetti *et al.*, 1989; Sorenson and Verbrugge, 1987). Evidence is now beginning to accumulate about both the positive and the negative effects of employment on women's health but most research has concentrated on major industries in the developed countries. As a result, the impact of waged work on millions of women in the formal and informal sectors of the global economy continues to go unrecorded and unregulated.

Most studies undertaken in the USA have been large-scale comparisons of the physical and mental health of women in employment with that of non-employed women. Most of these studies show that employed women as a group have better mental health than those remaining outside the labour market (Repetti *et al.*, 1989; Waldron and Jacobs, 1989). Similarly, most studies of physical health appear to demonstrate the positive effects of waged work.

The first health benefit for women entering the labour force is the financial reward it brings. Many give income as their prime motivation for employment and recent research in the UK suggests that at least four times more families than at present would be below the official poverty line if married women stopped going out to work (Glendinning and Millar, 1987, p. 6). In many parts of the third world the economic pressures are even greater as women are drawn into agricultural labour and plantation work in particular, but also industrial employment (Moore, 1988b, ch. 4). In the context of extreme poverty, income from waged work will usually offer significant health benefits to women and their families through the purchase of basic necessities such as housing and food. However, it is important to note that for some women, waged work may mean that long hours of labour keep them from tending family plots. Lack of food combined with overwork will then be damaging to their health (Mebrahtu, 1991; Raikes, 1989, p. 454).

Income from work outside the home can also enhance women's autonomy and hence their mental wellbeing through reducing their economic and social dependence on male partners. As one woman working in a Cairo factory expressed it:

> Work strengthens a women's position. The woman who works doesn't have to beg her husband for every piaster she needs. She can command respect in her home and can raise her voice in any decision (Ibrahim, 1985, quoted in Moore, 1988, p. 111).

But again, these potential benefits should not be overstated. Some women continue to be denied their right to autonomy and self-determination despite their economic contribution. In a recent study in a Punjab village, not one of the women interviewed said she alone could decide whether or not to work. Twenty-one out of twenty-nine said their husbands decided, three said their sons, and the rest mentioned other relatives. Only two said she and her partner would decide together. None could decide on how their wages would be spent (Horowitz and Kishwar, 1984, p. 95).

Finally, employment outside the home can be a source of companionship and provide a network of relationships to alleviate the isolation and feelings of worthlessness commonly expressed by some women at home (Warr and Parry, 1982; Brown and Harris, 1978). Recent American research suggests that the social support many women get from work is an important element in promoting both physical and mental health. Co-workers are often highly valued in this context, offering help with both domestic and work problems. Support of this kind seems to be especially beneficial to single mothers (Aneshensel, 1986; Repetti *et al.*, 1989, pp. 1398-9).

The potential benefits of waged work are therefore clear. But as we have seen, these benefits can be limited either by the domestic circumstances of the woman herself or by the nature of the job. Neither 'women' nor 'work' are homogeneous categories. Factors such as a woman's marital status, the domestic division of labour in her household, her age, the number of her dependents, her skills and her attitudes to employment will all affect the influence of work on her well-being, as will the nature of the job itself (Arber *et al.*, 1985). Hence large-scale studies comparing 'housewives' with women who are also employed outside the home can tell us very little either about the impact of work experiences on the health of different groups of women, or about sex differences in occupational health. The key question is not whether paid work in general is good for all women, but rather what the conditions are under which specific types of work will be harmful or beneficial for particular women in particular circumstances.

A detailed examination of women's role in the economy suggests that the physical and psychological hazards, which are not random, but reflect sexual divisions both in waged work and in the wider society. Nowhere in the world have women entered the labour force on equal terms with men. In most countries they are concentrated in particular sectors of the economy — in service jobs or in selected areas of manufacturing such as clothing and footwear, textiles, food processing and precision and electronic engineering. In most third world countries they make up a significant proportion of the labour force in agriculture. Within each area of work there is also a concentration of women in the jobs with lowest pay and least status. Thus, the labour market continues to be characterised by both horizontal and vertical segregation, with women's position being constrained by traditional notions about the sexual division of labour (*Feminist Review*, 1986; United Nations, 1991, pp. 87-8).

During the 1960s and 1970s, legislation was passed in the USA, Canada, Australia, and many European countries making it unlawful to pay women less than men for doing the same job, or to discriminate against them in selection and promotion (Meehan, 1985). However, women's earnings have not achieved parity with men's and they continue to be crowded into female 'employment ghettos' doing unskilled, monotonous jobs in shops, canteens, laundries, factories and hospitals. In most third world countries, the lack of any equal opportunities legislation means that women are entering employment under even less advantageous conditions. All over the world, women are more likely than men to work in small unregulated businesses, and are less likely to be members of trade unions.

It is also significant that much of the recent expansion of the female labour force has taken place among married women with children. Again, this pattern varies between countries, with ideologies of motherhood as well as the availability and cost of alternative sources of child care exerting an important influence. However, it is clear that mothers with dependent children form an increasingly large proportion of the world's labour force, fitting their hours around their children's needs and their domestic responsibilities, and often leaving little time for themselves. Though there is some evidence that the degree of inequality in the division of household labour is beginning to decrease — at least in the developed countries — employed women everywhere still retain primary responsibility for household work and this can have a serious effect on their well-being (Berk, 1985; Morris, 1990, ch. 5; United Nations, 1991, pp. 81–2).

Thus, sexual divisions, both in the home and in the workplace, continue to affect the impact of women's employment on their health. This will be explored in more detail through looking at a number of key issues. First, the physical hazards of the workplace which many women now share with men are examined. Second, the particular risks to women's reproductive systems generated by exposure to a variety of substances commonly used at work are explored. Third, the psychological stresses of work are examined in more detail, with particular reference to their relationship to the gendered nature of women's work. Finally, these three strands are drawn together through case studies of two classically 'female' jobs — nursing and clerical work.

Hazards of Waged Work

Many more women are now working in industry and are coming into contact with the sort of hazards some men (and a few women) have been facing for decades (WHO Regional Office for Europe, 1983). Women are increasingly exposed to hazardous chemicals, dusts, fumes and other toxic substances, as well as the physical strains of heavy labour. This is especially true in Eastern and South-eastern Asia where women now make up some 26 per cent of the manufacturing workforce (United Nations, 1991, p. 87). A brief account of the working life of one Indian woman serves to challenge any stereotype of weak and passive 'third world women'.

> Jayamma, a woman working for a brick kiln on the outskirts of Trivandrum, the capital of Kerala State, is almost fifty years old . . . As part of her equipment a woman brick-worker carries her own wooden plank, two feet by eight inches, to be used as a base on which to place the bricks . . . An adult woman carries twenty bricks, each weighing approximately one kilo, at a time. She must stack the bricks on her head by herself and carry them to the kiln, which may be ten or twenty minutes walk. The main brunt of the weight falls on her neck . . . And still these women virtually run . . . (Gulati, 1982, p. 361).

During the nineteenth century, many thousands of women in Europe, the USA, and India laboured in the unhealthy factories characteristic of the industrial revolution. For many, this carried on the traditional role of their mothers and grandmothers who had dominated the weaving trades before mechanisation (Lown and Chenut, 1983). Today, women workers still predominate in an industry which has been forced into a rapid restructuring to cope with recession. While the textile industry has shrunk in Europe, many thousands of women are still employed, often in depressed areas with a largely female and non-unionised labour force. In many under-developed countries women are entering textile factories in increasing numbers as multinational companies search the world for a cheap and 'docile' labour force (Chapkis and Enloe, 1983).

Yet work in the industry is still hazardous. Exposure to cotton dust can produce the debilitating respiratory disease byssinosis or 'brown lung'. In the early stages this leads to tightness in the chest, coughing and shortness of breath, and in the long run to severe congestion of the lungs and varying degrees of disability. Textile workers are also at risk from chemicals used in processing and dyeing the cloth, while garment workers are prone to accidents from needles. Formaldehyde, which is a suspected carcinogen, is widely used, as are other chemicals likely to produce allergies and industrial dermatitis. Textile mills are also notoriously noisy, making them stressful workplaces and sometimes inducing various degrees of deafness.

In the electronics industry, too, jobs are opening up for women both in the developed countries and in the third world. At first sight these factories appear to pose little risk to health. In practice, however, a great many hazards lie concealed from the needy and often unorganised women who flock to work in them. Worldwide, more than 50 per cent of workers on electronics production lines are women. In California's Silicon Valley, for instance, about 70,000 women are involved in the lowest levels of production, about 40 per cent of them Asians and Hispanics (Baker and Woodrow, 1984, p. 22). In other developed countries, electronics is expanding in areas of high unemployment, where traditional heavy industry has declined. The attraction of these 'enterprise zones' lies in the fact that they are able to offer employers tax concessions and investment grants as well as a reasonably compliant, largely female factory labour force.

In the third world, the benefits for employers are even greater, especially in Export Processing Zones (EPZs), with many governments offering tax exemption, free repatriation of profits, freedom from foreign exchange controls, and provision of loans at favourable rates of interest (Elson and Pearson, 1981; Lim, 1987; Lin, 1986; Mitter, 1986). In addition, most have little in the way of environmental controls or occupational health and safety regulation. As a result, electronics, like textiles, is increasingly moving toward South and South-east Asia and Latin America where the majority of workers in EPZs are now female (Mitter, 1986).

These developments do provide women with jobs in countries that traditionally offered them few opportunities for employment. However, there is growing evidence that many may be risking their health as a result (McCurdy *et al.*, 1989). A 1977 report from the US Occupational Health and Safety Administration put the scientific instruments industry and electrical equipment manufacturers first and third most hazardous amongst those industries exposing their workers to carcinogens (Baker and Woodrow, 1984, p. 25).

Despite growing epidemiological and toxicological evidence of hazards, there have been few studies of the health of workers in the electronics industry. Companies are secretive, materials are constantly changing, and the labour force has a high turnover rate making it difficult to exert pressure for investigation and regulation. However, formal evidence of neuropsychological damage to electronics workers is now beginning to emerge. In a comparison between a group of former electronics workers and a sample of matched controls, the former manifested inferior verbal ability, memory functions, visuospatial function, visuomotor speed, cognitive flexibility, psychomotor speed and reaction time and grip strength (Bowler *et al.*, 1991). The authors of the study attribute these findings to excessive solvent exposure and compare the effects to senile dementia. Women workers at the GTE Lenkurt plant in New Mexico experience them first hand every day:

> One woman said, 'My kids laugh at me. I used to keep a perfect house, and now they'll find the sugar bowl in the freezer. I put it

there'. Several women related getting lost on the freeway, which is difficult to do in Albuquerque because there are only two. Three had had the same experience — having to pull over and wait to remember where they had set out to go. Some of the stories come from husbands and children: mom is so out of it lately (Fox, 1991, p. 89).

Like the electronics industry, the agricultural sector, too, is often thought of as a safe workplace, providing labour in the open air and plenty of exercise. In reality, however, it can also pose a threat to women's health. According to official estimates, nearly 80 per cent of economically active women in sub-Saharan Africa, and at least half in Asia, are in agriculture (UN, 1991, p. 89). Many work extremely hard and in very harsh conditions and most female agricultural workers have no employment rights and little money. A research project carried out in Maharashtra, India, found a high incidence of stillbirths, premature births and deaths at the peak of the rice cultivation season. The work involves squatting and bending for hours leading to physical strain and pressure in the uterus.

It was a hot and humid late morning when I met Parvathi, eight months pregnant with her ninth child. She was on the top of a five feet high ladder tapping her 500 plus rubber trees. Tired, sweat glistening on her dark skin, Parvathi was panting as she spoke. She works for a contractor and therefore is not entitled to paid maternity leave. She will be back in the plantation a week after her delivery for her income is vital for the family's survival (Asian and Pacific Women's Resource Collection Network, 1989, p. 106).

Millions of women working on the land are also at risk from exposure to agrochemicals, many wrongly used and inadequately labelled. Again, the dangers are especially great in poorer parts of the world. According to an Oxfam study, there are at least 750,000 cases of accidental pesticide poisoning every year, with about 13,800 deaths worldwide, 10,000 of them in third world countries (Bull, 1982, p. 38). There are also chronic and long-term health effects such as cancers, birth defects and induced sterility for which no reliable data exist, while dust from rice husks can cause asthma, corneal scars and other eye problems (Asian and Pacific Women's Resource Collection Network, 1989, p. 105). We do not know how much of this damage is borne by women, but where they are substantially involved in agricultural production and/or live near the fields, they will inevitably figure prominently among the victims.

Since women are the lowest paid workers they often end up with the jobs no-one else wants to do and this frequently includes chemical spraying. Reports indicate that on Malaysian plantations about 80 per cent of those spreading herbicides are women (Ling, 1991, p. 23). They have little protective clothing or equipment when spraying highly toxic chemicals such as paraquat, which can cause damage to the lungs, heart, kidney, liver and central nervous system.

Reproductive Risks: Counting the Future Cost?

Concern that waged work would destroy women's capacity for successful motherhood was widespread during the nineteenth century in those countries where the industrial revolution brought more and more women into factory work. Indeed, it was concern for their children — both born and unborn — that provided the major impetus for the first phase of protective legislation enacted during the Victorian era. However, it was not until the latter part of the century that physical evidence of these risks began to emerge. In 1897, a study of 77 English females in the lead industry found that they had produced only 61 living children between them. Fifteen of the women had never become pregnant, there were 21 stillbirths and 90 miscarriages, and 40 of the 101 children born had died in their first year (Rom, 1976, p. 543). These early studies led several countries to implement special regulations prohibiting women from working in the lead industry, and these were later extended to other areas of employment. However, protective legislation has not solved the problem of exposure to reproductive hazards, either in the lead industry or elsewhere.

In many countries, evidence of reproductive hazards is ignored as women become ever more attractive as a labour force. Where action has been taken it has rarely involved changes in the workplace. Instead, protective legislation has been designed to stop women from working in conditions where they might endanger their offspring. Individual employers, too, have begun to exclude pregnant or potentially pregnant women to minimise their own liability should damage occur. Both the effectiveness and the equity of such strategies is being increasingly questioned as many women reject the idea that they should be forced to choose between employment and motherhood (Petchesky, 1979; Scott, 1984).

In 1978, five women employed at the Willow Island plant of the American Cynamid Corporation submitted to sterilisation in order to keep their jobs. A year earlier, the company had stated that all fertile women working in lead-exposed areas would have to be transferred to other tasks with lower earning potential or lose their job completely. This was to protect any unborn child from harm and to protect the company from possible law suits. Five of the women concerned chose sterilisation. As one explained: 'They don't have to hold a hammer to your head — all they have to do is tell you that's the only way you can keep your job' (Scott, 1984, p. 180).

At the same time, the introduction of equal rights legislation in many countries has led to doubts about the acceptability of protective legislation. In the United States, campaigning around this issue has been especially vigorous with women complaining that employers have seized upon protective legislation to exclude them from well-paid, traditionally male jobs just at the time when their legal rights were being extended (Bayer, 1982; Petchesky, 1979).

Women, Work and Stress: Adding Insult to Injury?

It is widely recognised that employment can also impose psychological costs. The conditions under which many women work have already been identified as stressful in studies of men: that is to say, they are in poorly paid, low status jobs which make high demands on them, but which offer little opportunity for control over their work. Factory jobs, for instance, often fit into this category, when they involve monotonous, uncreative, rigid tasks with a high level of supervision, sometimes including machine monitoring of output. Research has shown that such 'high strain' jobs can cause dissatisfaction and distress, and have a negative impact on men's health (Karasek, 1979; Karasek *et al.*, 1981; Karasek *et al.*, 1982). In the past few years, a number of studies have suggested that they may have the same effect on women (Haynes, 1991; Haynes *et al.*, 1987).

To this we have to add another potential stressor that is almost entirely a female experience: 'sexual harassment'. The scope of this distressing behaviour can be very broad, ranging from nude calendars on the wall through sexual jokes and propositions to unwanted touches and caresses and even rape. The vast majority of incidents involve women being harassed by men, very often those in a position of authority over them. As a result, many victims have to choose between sexual harassment and lack of promotion, low pay or even loss of their jobs. The sexual politics were made very clear at one clothing factory or 'maquiladora' on the Mexican American border:

> During the first years of the maquiladora program, sexual harassment was especially blatant. There were ingenieros who insisted on having only the prettiest women under their command. They developed a sort of factory 'harem'. Sandra knew of a man — 'would you believe this?' — who wanted as much female diversity as possible. All of the women on his crew, at his request had eyes and hair of a different color. Another man boasted that every women on his line had borne him a child (Fernandez Kelly, 1984: p. 241).

There has been little research on the impact of such experiences on the women involved. However, the Working Women's Institute in the USA has documented the health effects reported by women writing to them for help in harassment cases (Crull, 1984, p. 107). Nearly a half reported a deterioration in their work performance with many doubting their own abilities and even their career choice. Others reported that harassment exacerbated existing hazards, either because those involved were not concentrating properly, or because the men in question were deliberately behaving in a dangerous way. Virtually all the women reported at least one symptom of distress with anxiety, depression, anger, guilt and fear being most common.

We have seen that, contrary to popular belief, it is not only executives who suffer from work-related stress. In fact it is lower status jobs of the kind that most women occupy that appear to be particularly stressful. We can explore this in more detail through looking at two jobs — nursing and clerical work. Despite their 'soft' image both can expose women to both physical and psychological stressors.

Who Cares for Nurses?

About 90 per cent of all nurses are women. Nursing has been described as the most female of occupations, embodying the classic feminine virtues in their purest form. While the content of nursing will vary between societies, the universal element is care of those in need (Holden and Littlewood, 1991). Many women gain a great deal of satisfaction from this labour, but some will damage their own health in the process (Rogers and Salvage, 1988).

Nurses working in hospitals face hazards similar to those in industry, yet health and safety legislation has rarely been extended from the factory to the ward. Accidents are common in health work, especially those caused by lifting heavy patients. There are controls over the weight women can lift in industrial settings, and this has been used in the context of protective legislation to keep them out of areas like steel manufacture (Covell and Refshauge, 1986). However, no such regulations exist in the medical sector and there is often little help or appropriate equipment available. In the British context this is estimated to lead to the loss of at least 764,000 working days each year from back problems (Rogers and Salvage, 1988, p. 123).

Many nurses report puncture wounds and cuts (some of which may involve infection) while wet floors and crowded spaces can lead to a high injury rate, not just among nurses but among other women working in hospital kitchens and laundries. There is no accurate recording of these accidents but, according to the United States Department of Labor, occupational injury and illness is 55 per cent higher among hospital workers than among those in other service industries (Coleman and Dickinson, 1984, p. 44).

Nurses are also at risk from toxic chemicals. Antibiotics, detergents (such as hexachlorophene), disinfectants (especially formaldehyde) and sterilising fluids can all be a threat to health. They can lead to skin irritation or dermatitis and in some cases to more long-term problems. Therapeutic drugs such as penicillin and streptomycin are potential sensitisers that can eventually produce severe allergic reactions. Even more seriously, the cytotoxic drugs used to treat cancer patients can not only cause local toxic or allergic reactions, but are themselves carcinogenic and teratogenic. Yet adequate precautions are not always taken to protect those who administer them (Falk *et al.*, 1979). Anaesthetic gases can lead to headaches, irritability and depression, and have also been implicated in the causation of spontaneous abortions and birth defects (Edling, 1980; Vessey and Nunn, 1980). Finally, nurses may also be at risk from radiation. In many hospitals, records are kept of the exposure levels of radiologists and radiographers but not of nurses and other technicians. Thus, nursing can be a hard and dangerous job, as traditional risks such as infection are combined with the new hazards accompanying high technology medicine.

Nursing can also be psychologically stressful (Marshall, 1980; Smith, 1992). The task of caring for others can exert a powerful influence on women's mental health in both positive and negative ways. Different types of nursing vary in their psychological impact, with certain specialities involving more potentially stressful tasks than others. Different work settings will also have more or less supportive cultures. However, all nurses take on a significant degree of responsibility for managing the distress of others. This can be especially difficult when caring for people who are dying, for which many nurses report inadequate preparation and support.

Pam Smith has applied Arlie Hochschild's notion of emotional labour to nurses in an attempt to understand the nature of their work (Hochschild, 1983). She documents the way in which some nurses have to suppress very powerful feelings of their own in order to promote the well-being of those for whom they are caring:

> They think 'Oh yea, you're a nurse, you can manage'. But you can't really . . . Outwardly you might be managing, but you know I used to go home and cry my eyes out sometimes. It was dreadful. But I've found that at work you've almost got to be, well people expect you to be happy and not cross. And you can't be cross even though you feel like wringing someone's neck (Smith, 1992, p. 14).

The inevitable pressures of caring for others can be handled positively with appropriate training and support. However, they can also be extremely damaging as nurses struggle to maintain their own well-being. As one British psychiatric nurse said:

> We have no way of escaping . . . and sometimes if I've put a lot of effort in and they demand more and more then it begins to feel like 'You're taking my blood' — and it's not good to get into that position where you feel you've given someone a pound of flesh (Handy, 1991, p. 827).

Nurses are expected to take a great deal of responsibility for patient care but few have much control over their work. Too often they continue to be seen as the 'handmaidens' of doctors, with their working lives heavily supervised by nursing superiors, managers and medical staff (Gamarnikow, 1991; Game and Pringle, 1984, ch. 5; Salvage, 1985). Even where nurses' skills and knowledge are more extensive, they may have to 'defer' to those with higher status. A recent study of Canadian nurses found that the degree of control they had over their work was significantly associated with their job satisfaction and well-being (McLaney and Hurrell, 1988).

In many parts of the world, reductions in public expenditure over the last decade have increased the pressure on nurses. Both hospitals and community services are often understaffed, so that the pace of work is speeded up for individual nurses who feel unable to care adequately for their patients (Glazer, 1988). In Britain, the continuing financial constraints on the National Health Service have meant a damaging degree of overload for many nurses:

> Practical work conditions left me feeling pressured and stressed ... Ironically, it is because I wanted to remain 'caring' that I left nursing. Trying to care in the present system was a little like being flung in at the deep end with weights round my neck and told to swim. I think many nurses are in fact drowning, not waving, even if they have fixed smiles on their faces (*Medicine in Society*, 1983, p. 21).

Similar testimonies can be found from nurses in the USA:

> My first nursing job was on a forty bed medical ward in one of New York City's municipal hospitals. I had a lot of responsibility for my patients ... I quickly learned that unless my day was organised with clockwork routine and precise time allotments, I would soon fall behind. Then I would feel panic set in as things began to go wrong — an intravenous line that went dry, a medication error or omission, a forgotten promise to a patient ... I'd begin to cut corners, hoping that there would be no serious repercussions, that no-one would die, that no-one would find out ... (Coleman and Dickinson, 1984, p. 37).

The extent of the distress experienced by many nurses is evidenced by the very high rates of turnover and drop-out found in many countries. It was also demonstrated more formally in a study by the United States National Institute for Occupational Safety and Health (NIOSH). When 130 occupations were ranked according to their incidence of mental health problems, licensed practical nurses, nursing aides and registered nurses were ranked, 3, 10 and 27 respectively (Colligan *et al.*, 1977).

My Boss Gets On My Nerves: The Hidden Hazards of Office Work

Clerical work, too, can be stressful. In the United States this has been the fastest growing occupational category of the last decade. Some 80 per cent of clerical workers are women, and about one third of all women workers are in clerical jobs. Other industrialized countries show very similar trends, so that more women are now employed in offices than in any other type of workplace. Again, recent research has shattered complacency about 'female' jobs with the identification of significant physical hazards in what had been assumed to be a safe environment (Craig, 1981; Fleishman, 1984; Working Women's Education Fund, 1981). Offices are often ill designed and badly constructed, with little attention paid to the health of occupants. Unsuitable lighting, inadequate temperature and ventilation control, excessive noise and poorly constructed seating can all have deleterious effects on health, especially in the long term. There is also growing evidence of chemical hazards in the office. Solvents and correcting and cleaning fluids can cause dermatitis, eye and skin irritation, dizziness, headaches and allergic reactions. Some of the major correcting fluids contain perchloroethylene or 1.1.1 trichloroethane, which are suspected of causing cancer, while carbonless copy forms emit formaldehyde — an irritant and possible carcinogen (Fleishman, 1984).

Office machinery can also be hazardous to health. The use of photocopying machines involves exposure to several chemicals used mainly as cleaners and toners. Many of these are known to carry a significant risk if recommended exposure levels are exceeded (Stellman, 1977; Working Women's Education Fund, 1981). Some photocopying machines also emit ozone — a highly toxic gas that can cause nervous system, lung and genetic damage. Energy conservation policies have led to the tighter sealing of buildings, trapping chemical hazards inside. As a result, bacteria, dust, cigarette smoke and harmful chemicals all get recycled if there is inadequate ventilation. Although toxic exposures in offices usually occur at levels traditionally considered safe, the effects of very low level exposures over a working life are not yet understood.

In recent years, millions of women have also begun to use video display units (VDUs), often for a very high percentage of their working time (Westlander and Magnusson, 1988). For some, these machines have caused significant health problems (Henifin, 1984; Marschall and Gregory, 1983). Seven studies in the United States all found greater health problems among VDU users than among those not using the machines (Haynes, 1991, p. 161). There have been frequent reports of sore and tired eyes, prickling and burning sensations, twitching of the eye muscles and conjunctivitis. Staring at a VDU for many hours without sufficient breaks can also lead to nausea, headaches and digestive problems (Haynes *et al.*, 1987; Henifin, 1984).

VDU operators are one of the groups most likely to suffer from a syndrome that has come to be called Repetitive Strain Injury (RSI). This term came into use in Australia in the mid-1970s to describe the condition of workers suffering from pain and stiffness in particular muscles as a result of their repetitive use or the maintenance of constrained positions (London Hazards Centre, 1988; National Occupational Health and Safety Commission, 1986). Symptoms include fatigue, weakness, pain, muscle tightness, swelling and pins and needles. Feelings of frustration and depression also appear to be common, though the precise link between mental health and RSI needs further exploration. Significantly, RSI appears to be commonest among those who have least control over their work.

Many of those (predominantly women) with symptoms of RSI have experienced serious difficulties in getting their problems understood and accepted by doctors, causing further frustration and distress (Ewan *et al.*, 1991). As a result, the symptoms of RSI can affect all aspects of their life sending them on a 'pilgrimage of pain' in search of relief (Reid *et al.*, 1991).

As well as concerns about health problems resulting from using a VDU, there have also been concerns about the potential ill effects of simply being near the machines. Clusters of adverse reproductive outcomes have been reported in a number of different workplaces including the *Toronto Star Newspaper*, the Defence Logistics Agency and Southern Bell Telephone Company in Atlanta, and the public library in Aarhus, Denmark (De Matteo, 1985). Attempts to explore these further have come up with contradictory results.

Two Swedish studies found no relationship between VDU use and risk of miscarriage, and a study of 60,000 Canadian women had similar negative results (Erickson and Källen, 1986a and 1986b; McDonald *et al.*, 1986). However, recent research among 1,500 pregnant women in the United States found a significantly higher risk of miscarriage among those who reported using VDUs for more than twenty hours a week during the first three months of pregnancy (Goldhaber *et al.*, 1988). The debate over the possible reproductive risks of VDUs therefore remains unresolved. Further epidemiological research is needed with careful measurement of women's exposure. In the meantime, guidelines need to be designed and effectively implemented to ensure that women benefit from the new technologies without risking their health (Haynes, 1991, p. 166).

Although some women will move on from clerical and secretarial jobs to more senior positions, many are restricted to relatively low status jobs with little chance of promotion. They are often expected to take on considerable responsibility, but are not recognised or paid accordingly.

Again this 'job strain' appears to be reflected in their health. Research in the USA has shown that women in clerical jobs have significantly higher rates of coronary heart disease than other women (Haynes and Feinleib, 1980). Those most at risk had an unsupportive boss, lack of job change over a ten-year period, and difficulty in expressing anger. As the authors of one report on the health of office workers conclude:

> We now know that it is not only the highly paid executive who is likely to get a heart attack from the heavy responsibilities of his job. It is also his secretary. In fact an unsupportive boss may be hazardous to your health. (Working Women's Education Fund, 1981)

Conclusion

There is a complex relationship between women's waged work and their health. On the one hand, work outside the home can provide much needed material resources and the psychological benefits of improved status and greater independence, as well as important networks of social support. However, many women may have to purchase these benefits at the price of exposure to serious hazards, potential threats to their reproductive capacities, and considerable mental and physical distress. Any attempt to evaluate the health effects of waged work for women in particular communities will need to take these different elements into account.

It is also clear that waged work cannot be separated from the rest of women's lives. The boundaries of work and home are more permeable for women than for men and their mental and physical health will be moulded by their experiences as waged workers, parents and partners. Each type of activity will have its own effects, but they also have a collective influence. In some circumstances, the combination may be health-promoting as resources and support from one part of a women's life compensate for difficulties in another. However, in other circumstances it may create conflict and contradictions that are not conducive to health and well-being. As more women enter the labour force it becomes increasingly urgent for further research to clarify these issues so that policies can be designed to maximise the benefits and minimise the costs.

Note

Some material appearing in this chapter is also included in Doyal, L. (1995) *What Makes Women Sick? Gender and the Political Economy of Health*, London, Macmillan. An earlier version appeared in *Women's Studies International Forum* vol. 13, November 6 1990.

References

ANESHENSEL, C. (1986) 'Marital and employment role-strain, social support and depression among adult women' in HOBFOLL, S. E. (Ed.) *Stress, Social Support and Women*, New York, Hemisphere.

ARBER, S., GILBERT, N. and DALE, A. (1985) 'Paid employment and women's health: a benefit or a source of role strain?' *Sociology of Health and Illness*, **7**(3), 375–401.

ASIAN AND PACIFIC WOMEN'S RESOURCE COLLECTION NETWORK (1989) *Asian and Pacific Women's Resource and Action Series: health*, Kuala Lumpur, Asian and Pacific Development Centre.

BAKER, R. and WOODROW, S. (1984) 'The clean, light image of the electronics industry: miracle or mirage?' in: CHAVKIN, W. (Ed.) *Double Exposure? Women's Health Hazards on the Job and at Home*, New York, Monthly Review Press.

BAYER, R. (1982) 'Reproductive hazards in the workplace: bearing the burden of fetal risk', *Millbank Memorial Fund Quarterly*, **60**(4) 633–656.

BERK, S. (1985) *The Gender Factory: The Apportionment of Work in American Households*, New York, Plenum.

BOWLER, R., MERGLER, D., HUEL, G., HARRISON, R. and CONE, J. (1991) 'Neuropsychological impairment among former microelectronics workers', *Neurotoxicology*, **12**, 87–104.

BROWN, G. and HARRIS, T. (1978) *Social Origins of Depression*, London, Tavistock.

BULL, D. (1982) *A Growing Problem: Pesticides and the Third World Poor*, Oxford, Oxfam.

CHAPKIS, W. and ENLOE, C. (1983) *Of Common Cloth: Women in the Global Textile Industry*, Amsterdam, Transnational Institute.

CHAVKIN, W. (1984) *Double Exposure: Women's Health Hazards on the Job and at Home*, New York, Monthly Review Press.

CHESLER, P. (1972) *Women and Madness*, New York, Avon.

COLEMAN, L. and DICKINSON, C. (1984) 'The risks of healing: the hazards of the nursing profession', in CHAVKIN, W. (Ed.) *Double Exposure: Women's Health Hazards on the Job and at Home*, New York, Monthly Review Press.

COLLIGAN, M., SMITH, M. and HURRELL, J. (1977) 'Occupational incidence rates of mental health disorders', *Journal of Human Stress*, **3**, 34–39.

COVELL, D. and REFSHAUGE, C. (1986) 'Jobs for women challenges BHP: unmasking discriminatory safety practices', in *Proceedings of Conference: Women's Health in a Changing Society*, vol. 2, Adelaide, Australia, September 1985.

CRAIG, M. (1981) *The Office Workers' Survival Handbook*, London, British Society for Social Responsibility in Science.

CRULL, P. (1984) 'Sexual harassment and women's health', in CHAVKIN, W. (Ed.) *Double Exposure: Women's Health Hazards on the Job and at Home*, New York, Monthly Review Press.

DE MATTEO, B. (1985) *Terminal Shock: The Health Hazards of Video Display Terminals*. Toronto, NC Press.

EDLING, C. (1980) 'Anaesthetic gases as an occupational hazard – a review', *Scandinavian Journal of Work, Environment and Health*, **6**, 85–93.

EHRENREICH, B. and ENGLISH, D. (1979) *For Her Own Good: One Hundred and Fifty Years of the Experts' Advice to Women*, London, Pluto Press.

ELSON, D. and PEARSON, R. (1981) 'Nimble fingers make cheap workers: an analysis of women's employment in third world export manufacturing', *Feminist Review*, **7**, 87–107.

ERICSON, A. and KÄLLEN, B. (1986a) 'An epidemiology study of work with video screens and pregnancy outcome: I. registry study', *American Journal of Industrial Medicine*, **9**(5), 447–457.

ERICSON, A. and KÄLLEN, B. (1986b) 'An epidemiology study of work with video screens and pregnancy outcomes: II a case control study', *American Journal of Industrial Medicine*, **9**(5), 459–475.

EWAN, C. LOWY, E. and REID, J. (1991) 'Falling out of culture: the effects of repetition (*sic*) strain injury on sufferers' roles and identity', *Sociology of Health and Illness*, **13**(2), 168–192.

FALK, K., GORDON, P. and SORA, H. (1979) 'Mutogenicity in urine of nurses handling cytostatic drugs'. *Lancet*, **i** 1250–51.

Feminist Review, (1986) *Waged Work: a reader*, London, Virago.

FERNANDEZ KELLY, M. (1984) 'Maquiladoras: the view from inside', in SACKS, L. and REMY, D. (Eds) *My Troubles Are Going to Have Troubles With Me: Everyday Trials and Triumphs of Women Workers*, NJ, Rutgers University Press.

FLEISHMAN, J. (1984) 'The health hazards of office work', in CHAVKIN, W. (ed.) *Double Exposure: Women's Health Hazards on the Job and at Home*, New York, Monthly Review Press.

FOX, S. (1991) *Toxic Work: Women Workers at GTE Lenkurt*, Philadelphia, Temple University Press.

FRANKENHAUESER, M., LUNDBERG, U. and CHESNEY, M. (Eds) (1991) *Women, Work and Health: Stress and Opportunities*, New York, Plenum Press.

GAMARNIKOW, E. (1991) 'Nurse or woman: gender and professionalism in reformed nursing 1860–1923', in HOLDEN, P. and LITTLEWOOD, J. (Eds) *Anthropology and Nursing*, London, Routledge.

GAME, A. and PRINGLE, R. (1984) *Gender at Work*, London, Pluto Press.

GLAZER, N. (1988) 'Overlooked, overworked: women's unpaid and paid work in the health services "cost crisis"', *International Journal of Health Services*, **18**(1), 119–137.

GLENDINNING, C. and MILLER, J. (Eds) (1987) *Women and Poverty in Britain*, Brighton, Harvester.

GOLDHABER, M., POLEN, M. and HIATT, R. (1988) 'The risk of miscarriage and birth defects among women who use visual display terminals during pregnancy', *American Journal of Industrial Medicine*, **13**, 695–706.

GULATI, L. (1982) *Profiles in Female Poverty: A Study of Five Women Workers in Kerala*, London, Pergamon Press.

HANDY, J. (1991) 'The social context of occupational stress in a caring profession', *Social Science and Medicine*, **32**(7), 819–830.

HAYNES, S. (1991) 'The effect of job demands, job control and new technologies on the health of employed women: a review', in FRANKENHAUESER, M., LUNDBERG, U. and CHESNEY, M. (Eds) *Women, Work and Health: Stress and Opportunties*. New York, Plenum Press.

HAYNES, S. and FEINLEIB, M. (1980) 'Women, work and coronary heart disease: prospective findings from the Framingham Heart Study', *American Journal of Public Health*, **70**, 113–141.

HAYNES, S., LaCROIX, A. and LIPPIN, T. (1987) 'The effect of high job demands and low control on the health of employed women', in QUICK, J. BHAGAT, R., DALTON, J. and QUICK, J. (Eds) *Work, Stress and Health Care*, New York, Praeger.

HENIFIN, M. S. (1984) 'The particular problems of video display terminals', in CHAVKIN, W. (Ed.) *Double Exposure: Women's Health Hazards on the Job and at Home*. New York, Monthly Review Press.

HOCHSCHILD, A. (1983) *The Managed Heart: Commercialisation of Human Feeling*. San Francisco, University of California Press.

HOLDEN, P. and LITTLEWOOD, J. (1991) *Anthropology and Nursing*, London, Routledge.

HOROWITZ, S. and KISHWAR, M. (1984) 'Family Life: the unequal deal', in KISHWAR, M. and VANITA, R. (Eds) *In Search of Answers: Indian Women's Voices from Manushi*, London, Zed Books.

IBRAHIM, B. (1985) 'Cairo's factory women', in FERNEA, E. (Ed.) *Women and the Family in the Middle East*, Austin, University of Texas Press.

KARASEK, R. (1979) 'Job demands, job decision latitude and mental strain: implications for job redesign', *Administrative Science Quarterly*, **24**, 285–308.

KARASEK, R., BAKER, D., MARXER, F., AHLBLOM, A. and THEORELL, T. (1981) 'Job decision latitude, job demands and cardiovascular disease: a prospective study of Swedish men', *American Journal of Public Health*, **71**(7), 694–705.

KARASEK, R., RUSSELL, R. and THEORELL, T. (1982) 'Psychology of stress and regeneration in job-related cardiovascular illness', *Journal of Human Stress*, **8**(March), 29–42.

LIM, L. (1978) *Women Workers in Multinational Corporations: the case of the electronics industry in Malaysia and Singapore*, Michigan University Occasional Papers no. IX, Fall.

LIN, V. (1986) *Health, Women's Work and Industrialisation: women workers in the semiconductor industry in Singapore and Malaysia*, Working Paper no. 130, Michigan State University, Women in International Development.

LING, C. (1991) 'Women and the environment: the Malaysian experience', in WALLACE, T. and MARCH, C. (Eds) *Changing Perceptions: Writings on Gender and Development*, Oxford, Oxfam.

LONDON HAZARDS CENTRE (1988) *Repetition Strain Injury: hidden harm from overuse*, London, London Hazards Centre Trust.

LOWN, J. and CHENUT, H. (1983) 'The patriarchal thread — a history of exploitation', in CHAPKIS, W. and ENLOE, C. (Eds) *Of Common Cloth: Women in the Global Textile Industry*, Amsterdam, Transnational Institute.

McCURDY, S. A., SCHENKER, M. and LASSITER, D. (1989) 'Occupational injury and illness in the semiconductor manufacturing industry', *American Journal of Industrial Medicines*, **15**(5), 499–510.

McDONALD, A. D., CHERRY, N., DELORME, C. and McDONALD, J. (1986) 'Visual display units and pregnancy: evidence from the Montreal Survey', *Journal of Occupational Medicine*, **28**(12), 1226–1231.

McLANEY, H. and HURRELL, J. (1988) 'Control, stress and job satisfaction in Canadian nurses', *Work and Stress*, **3**, 217–224.

MARSCHALL, D. and GREGORY, J. (1983) *Office Automation: Jekyll or Hyde?*, Cleveland, Ohio, Working Women Education Fund.

MARSHALL, J. (1980) 'Stress amongst nurses', in COOPER, C. and MARSHALL, J. (Eds) *White Collar and Professional Stress*, John Wiley & Sons.

MEBRAHTU, S. (1991) 'Women, work and nutrition in Nigeria', in TURSHEN, M. (Ed.) *Women and Health in Africa*, Trenton, NJ, Africa World Press.

Medicine in Society (1983) Special issue on nurses and nursing: **8**(4), 14–35.

MEEHAN, E. (1985) *Women's Rights at Work: Campaigns and Policy in Britain and the United States*, London, Macmillan.

MITTER, S. (1986) *Common Fate, Common Bond: Women in the Global Economy*, London, Pluto Press.

MOORE, H. (1988) *Feminism and Anthropology*, Oxford, Polity Press.

MORRIS, L. (1990) *The Workings of the Household*, Oxford, Polity Press.

NATIONAL OCCUPATIONAL HEALTH AND SAFETY COMMISSION (1986) *Repetitive Strain Injury: A Report and Model Code of Practice*, Canberra, Australian Government Publishing Service.

PETCHESKY, R. (1979) 'Workers, reproductive hazards and the politics of protection: an introduction', *Feminist Studies*, **5**(Summer) 233–245.

RAIKES, A. (1989) 'Women's health in East Africa', *Social Science and Medicine*, **28**(5), 447–459.

REID, J., EWAN, C. and LOWY, E. (1991) 'Pilgrimage of pain: the illness experiences of women with repetitive strain injury and the search for credibility', *Social Science and Medicine*, **32**(5), 601–612.

REPETTI, R., MATTHEWS, K. and WALDRON, I. (1989) 'Employment and women's health: effects of paid employment on women's mental and physical health', *American Psychologist*, **44**(11), November, 1394–1401.

ROGERS, R. and SALVAGE, J. (1988) *Nurses at Risk: A Guide to Health and Safety at Work*, London, Heinemann.

ROM, W. (1976) 'Effects of lead on the female and reproduction: a review', *Mount Sinai Journal of Medicine*, **43**(5), 542–52.

SALVAGE, J. (1985) *The Politics of Nursing*, London, Heinemann.

SCOTT, J. (1984) 'Keeping women in their place: exclusionary policies and reproduction', in CHAVKIN, W. (Ed.) *Double Exposure: Women's Health Hazards on the Job and at Home*, New York, Monthly Review Press.

SMITH, P. (1992) *The Emotional Labour of Nursing: How Nurses Care*, London, Macmillan.

SORENSEN, G. and VERBRUGGE, L. (1987) 'Women, work and health'. *American Review of Public Health*, **8**, 235–51.

STELLMAN, J. (1977) *Women's Work, Women's Health: Myths and Realities*, New York, Pantheon.

UNITED NATIONS (1991) *The World's Women: trends and statistics 1970–1990*. UN, New York.

VESSEY, M. and NUNN, J. (1980) 'Occupational hazards of anaesthesia', *British Medical Journal*, **281**, 696–98.

WALDRON, I. and JACOBS, J. (1989) 'Effects of labor force participation on women's health: new evidence from a longitudinal study', *Journal of Occupational Medicine*, **30**, 977–983.

WARR, P. and PARRY, G. (1982) 'Paid employment and women's psychological wellbeing', *Psychological Bulletin*, **91**(3), 498–516.

WESTLANDER, G. and MAGNUSSON, B. (1988) 'Swedish women and new technology', in WESTLANDER, G. and STELLMAN, J. (Eds) *Women and Health*, **13**, New York, Haworth Press.

WORKING WOMEN'S EDUCATION FUND (1981) *Warning: Health Hazards for Office Workers*, available from Working Women's Education Fund, 1224 Huron Road, Cleveland, Ohio 44115.

WORLD HEALTH ORGANISATION, REGIONAL OFFICE FOR EUROPE (1983) *Women and Occupational Health Risks*, EURO Reports and Studies, 76, Copenhagen.

Chapter 6

What Can She Depend On? Substance Use and Women's Health

Elizabeth Ettorre

As a feminist scholar who for fifteen years has studied women's use of substances, I have found addiction professionals, whether they are researchers or clinicians, male or female, to be deeply resistant to the need for a feminist perspective in this area of study. Given this deep level of resistance, two very basic ideas need to be injected into this field if a feminist perspective is to develop. First, we need to be relatively familiar with the social scientific way of viewing the world and in particular, with how the notion of gender has had an impact on recent developments in the sociology of health and illness. Second, we need to be open, both theoretically and methodologically, to an approach which is sensitive to the needs of women as a social group.

Until these ideas are recognised as important, it is difficult to see how addiction studies will facilitate the creation of an intellectual environment in which the production of feminist knowledge is a real possibility. Within the addiction field, as in other related fields of health research, there is a need for a sound theoretical framework challenging traditional research practices which are gender biased, gender blind and one-dimensional (Ettorre and Riska, 1993). Therefore, a major strand of thinking throughout this chapter is that a women sensitive response rooted in the identity and consciousness of women substance users is essential.

This chapter is divided into two sections. In the first section, key issues which relate to women and substance use as a feminist issue are outlined. After looking at the need to develop a feminist framework, four related issues in the establishment of a feminist perspective in this field are examined. These include: the importance of the concept 'substance use'; the implications of using, what I call a dual conception of dependency; developing a feminist methodology; and linking pleasure to this area of study.

In the second section, the potential for effective social action *vis-à-vis* women substance users is discussed. Looking at ideas behind the development of a feminist epistemology in this area, the types of feminist strategies needed both collectively and individually for women substance users to achieve increased visibility and effectiveness are examined.

Here, I offer a viewpoint which can be viewed as both integrative and empowering rather than rhetorical or polemical. Although what follows tends to raise questions rather than to provide 'pat' answers, it is a sincere attempt to look at a well-established area of study in a different light. For example, my contention throughout this chapter is that previous work in this field offers little if any insight into the interplay between the public and the private spheres of the lives of women substance users. In this way, the critical perspective put forward should stimulate useful issues for further debate.

Key Issues

Moving from 'Masculinist' to Feminist Ways of Thinking

Drugs have distinct social spaces in diverse cultures; they are most definitely substances affecting human behaviour. Drugs have symbolic value and culturally based meanings which influence expectations of effects and actual experience of drug taking (Bruun *et al.*, 1975, p. 4). Nevertheless, regardless of the culture, society or defined social space in which they find themselves, women substance users will experience not only their drugs as having a symbolic value but also themselves as being symbols of deviant and marginal women. Drug use is emblematic of their failure as women.

It is fair to say that most research in the addiction field ignores the above, important issues. As a result, the significance of substance use for women as a social group is more often than not subverted. By centring on men, the most socially visible participants within our drug using cultures, scientific research upholds traditional, partiarchal[1] images of men and women. It is almost as if drugs 'naturally' belong to men. In effect, a distorted view of gender is presented. Here, I contend that the development of a feminist analysis, similar to the critique offered within the area of science and technology, would be useful in order to provide a more balanced picture. Only then could we move effectively beyond, what Rose (1986) calls, 'masculinist realities' and challenge patriarchal notions, oppressive to women.

Within the field of addiction, the centrality of these traditional notions (i.e. men as socially dominant and active participants in the drug using culture, and women as socially subordinate and relatively passive participants) has meant that the situations and needs of women were largely unacknowledged within both the treatment and research world. In this context, Holstein (1987) has shown how experts in the general mental health field produce 'gender laden rhetoric' in their diagnostic practice. I would suggest further that gender-laden rhetoric is also rampant in the addiction field.

The difficulties of introducing critical work on gender as a valid area for research should not be under-emphasised. Indeed, the study of women and addiction has been referred to as a 'non-field', although the impact of the Women's Liberation Movement has been recognised by some as an important catalyst for change in this area (Kalant, 1980). The lack of a body of knowledge about women and substance use led those working in the field, specifically psychiatrists and psychologists, to assume that substance use was primarily a 'man's disease' or a 'male problem'. Women were effectively ignored and excluded from these analyses.

While feminist researchers and those sympathetic to a feminist approach have placed women firmly within the addiction field (Bepko, 1991; Sargent, 1992; Ettorre, 1989a, 1992), the model of traditional research functions to disempower women in the field (Forth-Finegan, 1991). Although I have already outlined elsewhere (Ettorre, 1986) with special reference to alcohol sociology, strategies necessary for the establishment of a feminist perspective, I should emphasize that in this context also this involves a new way of seeing, and the transformation of traditional views into what I would call a gender-sensitive perspective. This perspective reflects the somewhat invisible realities of women's every day lives.

Let us now explore four key issues related to the development of a feminist perspective: substance use; dependency; feminist methodology; and pleasure.

The importance of the concept 'substance use'
To gain a full insight into a feminist issue such as substance use, we need to be aware that there are many social complexities that are not apparent at first glance. We need to unearth the genealogy of women's collective

survival vis-à-vis dependency producing or addictive substances. Simply, we need to discover our particular herstories, reflecting the constant struggle for women to maintain our female integrity and self-worth in substance abusing, stress-filled societies. That Western industralized countries are societies dependent economically, politically and culturally on a cushioning process, provided by a variety of chemical comforts, indicates the extent to which addiction (and indeed stress) have become 'normal', established facts of life. The irony associated with this sort of cultural process is that chemical comforts or drugs can provide only temporary relief (Gossop, 1982). None of these substances is able to solve the normal problems of living and for women, the notion, 'problems of living', has specific social and cultural ramifications.

Since the late 1970s, women researchers in the field have looked at the consequences of 'a tranquilliser trap for women' (Melville, 1984); 'women bottling it up' (Curran and Golombok, 1985); 'cigarettes as ladykillers' (Jacobson, 1981, 1986); 'women under the influence' (McConville, 1983); 'the stigma attached to women alcoholics' (Beckman, 1978); 'the female junkie' (Perry, 1979; Rosenbaum, 1981); and even 'women's abuse of food as a social disease' (Orbach, 1978). From this work, women were viewed as abusers of a whole series of substances and they were portrayed as either out of control, in need of control, or both. These women researchers speculated that unless these powerful notions were confronted and indeed challenged, there was a danger that those responding to women in need of help could unknowingly perpetuate myths and stereotypes, harmful to the healing process. More recent research, again by women, has outlined in detail the wounds inflicted on women substance users during the supposed healing process of official treatment (Mason, 1991); by the cultural imperative targeting women as carriers of shame (Miller, 1991) and in the process of self-recovery (Hafner, 1992).

From the above, we may already sense that the majority of discussions about women within the addiction field focus primarily on substances which are 'mind altering'. Reflecting on the context of these discussions, I would argue that the terms 'addiction' or 'drug use' do not mirror adequately women's somewhat problematic relationship to substances, regardless of whether or not they are 'mind altering'. For example, there has been a growing body of feminist literature looking at the consequences of women's use and abuse of food (Orbach, 1978; Chernin, 1981, 1985; Lawrence, 1987; Bovey, 1989; Hirshman and Munter, 1989). Although anorexia nervosa and bulimia nervosa exist as diagnostic categories for both men and women, the terms 'anorexics' and 'bulimics' tend to conjure up images of emaciated, self-starving women, while most anorexics and bulimics are women. In this context, Orbach (1986, p. 24) argues quite convincingly that as key features of anorexia, 'the starvation amidst plenty, the denial set against desire, the striving for invisibility versus the wish to be seen are a metaphor for our age'. Furthermore, women's problematic relationship with food may be seen as an excruciating spectacle in which women actually 'transform their bodies' in an attempt to deal with the contradictory requirements of the contemporary female role.

Given the above discussion, it appears that substance use is a more useful notion than the traditional terms 'addiction' or 'drug use'. Substance use, as a more inclusive notion for women, provides the necessary conceptual foundation upon which a feminist perspective can be built. Within the addiction field, this notion helps to clarify outdated theoretical boundaries, which need to be expanded if a full understanding of women and substance use is to become a reality. The underlying assumption here is that we cannot adequately comprehend the problems faced by women dependent on substances such as alcohol, prescribed drugs, illicit drugs, cigarettes, foods, etc., without knowledge which is rooted in our experiences as women. Here, I would argue that within this vast area of women's reality, a feminist perspective as well as a clear, women-orientated response rooted in the identity and consciousness of women substance users are essential.

Let us now look at how, for women, the notion of substance use may also imply varying levels of dependency on a variety of substances, and at how this notion can be linked with a general, feminist issue: dependency.

Using a dual conception of dependency

A very basic fibre of feminist thought is the idea that women, more than men, are socialised into dependency. In earlier contexts (Ettorre, 1989a, 1989b, 1992), I have discussed a dual conception of dependency with special reference to women and substance use. In these discussions, I have outlined the subtle implications of this dual conception for women substance users as a social group. I summarise this work below. Looking at the etymological roots of dependency, we find that dependency has two meanings: 'addiction' and 'a subordinate thing'. Making a distinction between these two definitions, I have called the former definition dependency of the 'addiction' kind, and the latter dependency of the 'subordinate thing' kind. For women as a social group, the former definition (dependency of the addiction kind) is the unacceptable face of dependency, while the latter meaning (dependency of the subordinate thing kind) is not only the acceptable face of dependency, but also the prescribed norm.

For example, dependency of the addiction kind is socially unacceptable because it is seen to interfere with a women's social role as housewife, mother, dutiful daughter or female worker. On the other hand, dependency of the subordinate thing kind is seen to be good, highly valued or socially acceptable because it involves being dependent on a male partner, male protectors or male superiors. The relations of patriarchy and female dependency seem to go hand in hand. The acceptable face of dependency is not only viewed as a fundamental part of any woman's life but it is the central operating principle in her life, her *raison d'être*. Gloria Steinem (1979, p. 66) has gone so far as to suggest that all women are 'male junkies', that is 'people who need regular shots of male-approval and presence both professionally and personally'.

But there is another side to this issue which complicates matters. Over the years, feminist thinkers (Graham, 1983; Finch and Groves, 1982) have demonstrated that women's dependent status is contingent upon their being, at the same time, depended upon by others. Indeed this is a growing interest within mainstream sociology. (See for example, Giddens, 1992, pp. 87–110). In other words, dependency not only involves a cycle of caring, but, in turn, this cycle involves caring work which is obviously gendered work but also, more often than not, health related (Graham, 1990). Therefore, for many women, involvement in the social organisation of caring implies giving care and helping others. This is a fundamental part of the process of being dependent.

In this light, we can see that dependency has various shades of meanings on both a public and a private level. This suggests that a thorough enquiry into the women and substance use issue needs to highlight key individual and social factors. Simply, we need to offer a full account of the day-to-day experiences of these women. We need much more work in this area by women and for women. Now, I will turn to feminist methodology.

Developing a feminist methodology
This section highlights the problems that exist within the traditional research framework on women and substance use. In order to build up a feminist perspective in this area, we first need to be aware of four problems.

First, traditional research tends to view women substance users as an homogeneous group. There is little if any reference to key social factors such as age, ethnic origins, race, social class, sexual orientation, and their effects on experience. To challenge traditional accounts we need to extend our analysis within and beyond established treatment settings and to challenge traditional research environments, 'taken for granted' social groupings, particular academic disciplines and specific cultures. Given that we live in societies characterised by a vast range of social inequalities, we should assess how these inequalities affect our own research practices.

If we want to expand our work by focusing on specific groups of women such as working-class women, black women, women from different ethnic minorities, lesbian women or single women, we need to examine social attitudes and practices furthering inequalities in the class system, institutionalised racism, heterosexism, or social arrangements detrimental to single parents. While much sociological research has been done on the family, feminist research which emphasizes the effects of women's substance use on the interplay between the public, primary sphere of social relations and the private, secondary sphere of social relations is badly needed.

Second, traditional research in this area tends to individualise the issue of substance use for women. This type of focus has distorted the image of women substance users. My contention is that the area needs a vibrant analysis inclusive of what I call *both* the 'structural' and the 'processual' approach. For example, I would contend that a processual approach focusing primarily on the individual and/or on female help seekers is quite limited. (See for example, Thom, 1984, 1986, 1987; Allan, 1987). While this approach helps us to get at subtle (and often hidden) subjective meanings of substance use, this perspective remains generally uncritical and ahistorical. More specifically, it is unable to explain fully the structural roots of power. And for women, the issue of power (whether cultural, social, political or economic) is of crucial importance: see for example, Kitzinger (1991).

If a feminist approach is to develop in this area, clear links between the issue of women and substance use and the overall structural dynamics of power and dependency must be established. Here, I use the term 'feminist approach' because there is a vast difference between offering analyses based on an uncritical acceptance of women's role, gender arrangements, patriarchal power, and so on, and proposing theories and explanations grounded in women-orientated frameworks. Work on women and substance use is not necessarily feminist simply because it focuses on women. If the central principle upholds the image of women substance abusers as helpless 'victims'; if the topic is introduced in a distorted or gender-insensitive way, the subordination of women remains unchallenged. Furthermore, in this kind of work the social order of the established gender divisions is denied, and the feminist notion that 'the private/female sphere is dependent on the public/male sphere' (Garmarnikow *et al.*, 1983) may be totally hidden. Breaking away from the traditional framework, we, as feminists, need to highlight women's collective experiences. We need to ask why some women seek lifestyles and behaviours that damage their health. (See also Graham, this volume.) A collective focus enhances a political awareness.

Third, traditional research frameworks tend to have an elevated view of 'treatment'. In other words, treatment is viewed as an exalted end in itself or as the highest form of institutionalised care for substance users, rather than as a powerful but imperfect resource within society. We need a pragmatic approach to treatment (MacGregor and Ettorre, 1987), which views treatment as a means to an end, as well as a visible way of catering to the special needs of all clients. In this way, the concept of difference is incorporated within a treatment structure, and services become more flexible in response to the needs of specific groups (e.g. women with children, members of the black community, the unemployed, single parents, and so on). Such 'difference-sensitive' treatment provides an holistic approach, offering an insider's sensitivity to women's problems.

Fourth, as conscientious scholars we need to consider ways of extending our analyses beyond traditional research frameworks into wider social arenas. For example, Graham's work on women's smoking (Graham, 1987; and this volume) demonstrates quite effectively how the issue of women and substance use can be linked with wider health and welfare concerns such as poverty, single parenthood, family health and leisure. More broadly, within the field of substance use, a feminist perspective (Ettorre, 1992; Bepko, 1991) including an interest in the specificities of age, ethnic origins, preferred drug, sexual preference and cultural settings (Wolfson and Murray, 1987; Ettorre, forthcoming; Gefou-Madianou, 1992) is beginning to develop.

In looking at these four limitations of the traditional research frameworks, I have established pointers for the development of a feminist methodology in this field. Beyond this, traditional research frameworks are amenable to expansion and transformation through the adoption of a feminist perspective. In the following discussion, I introduce the concept of pleasure into this research arena and explore the relevance of this concept for women substance users as a social group.

Linking pleasure to this area of study
When the problems of women substance users are taken out of the private domain, 'experts' more often than not fail to see the variety of reasons why women use drugs *differently* from men. Women's substance abuse is seen as more of a social problem than men's because it implies instability in the family. For example, images of the woman who abuses alcohol have been experienced historically as a real threat to the clear lines between the gender roles of men and women (Appel, 1990; van Nieuwkerk, 1992). Furthermore, there are few public settings, contexts or mechanisms whereby women substance users can address their experiences in terms of the choices they make or the benefits they receive from their consumption of addictive substances. Underlying their substance use is the type of voluntary, active and creative use of drugs which Harpwood (1982) describes and illustrates so well. (See also Graham, this volume.)

In discussing the concept of pleasure, I am not advocating substance abuse. Rather I am suggesting that we need to look more closely at the pleasurable effects of substances and in particular, to see why and how women experience their substance use as pleasurable. A possible starting point is to ask: 'what pleases women'? We already know that the concept of pleasure for both men and women tends to be linked with sexual performance and pursuits and that in the sexual arena, male sexual dominance is assumed to be 'natural' (Holland *et al.*, 1990; Thomson and Holland, this volume). However, pleasure has other meanings that extend beyond the realm of the sexual. As Raymond (1986) suggests, pleasure for women includes the notion of empowerment. Furthermore, it has been demonstrated that pleasure and empowerment are linked particularly for those in a subordinate, social position: i.e. women (Vance, 1984). I would also suggest that women's experience of pleasure is closely related to their specific material circumstances and life-style choices (i.e. age, social class, sexual orientation, relationship status, ethnic origins, psychological health, physical well-being, accommodation, number of dependants, paid employment, and so on).

Given this view, pleasure for most women appears only as a hidden reality, subverted by oppressive social structures. To break from these structures women need to become grounded in the positive dimensions of what Raymond (1986) calls their otherness. The observation that some women turn to substances for pleasurable experiences could be an indication of this grounding process. For example, it has been suggested that for women 'taking drugs can be an attempt to meet our own needs' (Dawn, 1986). Do women turn to substances as a way of taking something for themselves, rather than giving and receiving pleasure as is the usual case? Here, pleasure implies a certain amount of autonomy.

In the context of feminist theory, Daly (1984) contends that many women, because of their fragmented and isolated lives, accept the belief that happiness is attainable only after death. In an attempt to counter this belief, Daly urges women to recognise that their quest for pleasure or 'lust for happiness' is a quest for a life of activity. In the highest sense, this life of activity is contemplation or an activity of the mind. Here, Daly is not proposing that all women should leave secular society and enter the reflective world of the cloister. Rather, she is suggesting that 'women's whole, intellectual/passionate/sentient selves need to unfold' (Daly, 1984, p. 347) as women become pleasure seekers. (Of course, this appears only as an option for relatively privileged women.)

This distinctly feminist process demands that we become deeply in touch with our creative powers; recognise our integrity as women and most importantly, develop ways of resisting and perhaps transcending patriarchal patterns of thinking, speaking and acting. Women need more public and private space to explore what pleases us and to empower ourselves as women. Specifically, women substance users need to explore the many and often contradictory, reasons why they use substances. They need to challenge stereotypical images which characterise them as diseased, neurotic, pathological, decadent or polluted and assert their own realities.

The above discussions have helped to generate an awareness of the need for a feminist perspective in the field of substance use. The following section examines the potential for effective social action *vis-à-vis* women substance users. Here, my basic assumption is that women's praxis, while existing in seed form, needs to be nurtured, encouraged and developed. I ask: What types of feminist strategies[2] are needed, both collectively and individually, for women substance users to achieve increased visibility and effectiveness?

Key Strategies

Women's Praxis and Women's Health: Developing a Feminist Epistemology

The generation of a feminist awareness of women and substance use has identifiable roots in the women's health movement, based on the need for a collective, social approach to the problems of women's ill health. This movement has consistently emphasised the need for women's self-help, women-centred health education, women-centred health care provision and campaigns around specific feminist health care issues. Women's praxis is focused on developing strategies which ensure women's physical as well as emotional well-being, using a strategic approach which aims to abolish obstacles to the achievement of a more caring, humane approach to women's health.

While individually-focused medicine does not consider the social origins of many illnesses, the women's health movement has attempted to do so. Rather than blame ourselves for ill health, we can see that damaging social experiences may produce ill health and furthermore, remedial action needs to be social (Thunhurst, 1982).

Feminist social action in the health field is about changing consciousness, providing appropriate health-related services and struggling to change established health institutions (Fruchter *et al.*, 1977). It is also about educating ourselves to see that the control of our health and fertility is fundamental to the control of our lives (Boston Women's Health Collective, 1978). Here, the implication is that medicine is more than a servicing profession: it is an institution of social control. Furthermore, women need to understand their oppression at the hands of the medical profession before they can change it. In this way, the women's health movement has been a real challenge to male professional authority (Ruzek, 1978).

Reflecting on the origins of feminist health activism, Lesley Doyal (1983) outlines the historical stages of the British women's health movement and focuses on the concept of reproduction (both ideological and biological) as a useful one in explaining the relationship between women and medicine. She argues that on the ideological level, 'medical knowledge and practice are part of the means by which gender divisions in society are maintained' (p. 379). Medicine is deeply involved in the reproduction of a specific view of the intrinsic character of women. In effect, medicine does not invent our social roles, it merely interprets them to women as biological destiny (Ehrenreich and English, 1974).

Clearly, the relationship between women's bodies, biological reproduction and medicine is an oppressive one in which women lose out. While Doyal (1983) is aware that medicine plays a part in the overall reproduction of the relations of production, she also recognises the importance of its control over biological reproduction. Simply, medical control over female reproduction upholds existing gender, class, and indeed race relations. Furthermore, Doyal and Elston (1986, p. 202) argue that within a feminist critique of medicine, women have generated political responses focused on four key areas of activity: 're-defining women as healthy; overcoming women's ignorance; attacking sexist beliefs and practices; and seizing the means of reproduction for themselves'.

In the light of the above and with special reference to the substance use field, it could be argued that the issue of women and substance use has become more visible from within traditional self-help groups (NA, AA, ACOA, Overeaters Anonymous, Weight Watchers, etc.) than from the WLM or specifically, the women's health movement. Although a feminist analysis of substance use exists in seed form in the WLM, a greater awareness of the dual notions of dependency needs to be generated in order to challenge the dominance of traditional self-help groups in this area, and it is fair to say that the areas of activity mentioned above remain 'under-developed', if not undeveloped.

Developing Feminist Strategies: We Need a Creative Response

Hopefully, there is now an awareness that issues relating to women and substance use benefits from an injection of feminist politics, and a clear women-orientated approach. In the above discussion, I established the groundwork for this type of politics. Here, I contend that specific strategies are needed for the increased attention to the women and substance use issue within the women's health movement. These strategies include: developing social agency; seeing pollution as a political issue; and publicising pain as well as pleasure.

Developing social agency
Women substance users need to be acutely aware that 'it is not enough to move women away from danger and oppression; it is necessary to move toward something: toward pleasure, agency, self-definition' (Vance, 1984, p. 24). 'Moving towards something' is a feminist process already proven successful in the women and health field (Ernst and

Maguire, 1987), whereby women develop separate, strong identities within a collective framework. For women substance users, this strategy could become a fundamental part of their self-help and feminist practice. Indeed, there is a need for a collective context in which women are able to re-affirm their identity as women and to reject, whole-heartedly, the labels 'junkie'; 'food addict', 'alcoholic' or 'tranx addict'.

In developing social agency, women need to recognise that they are what Lewin (1985, p. 125) refers to as 'strategic actors'. The strategies revealed in the ways women use substances are not individually-specific but reveal common patterns of experience. It could be argued that women, as strategic actors, choose to use substances as a way of adjusting or modifying their behaviour in response to their oppressive social situations. In this light, their choice is perceived as creative, if not empowering. In other words, it is perceived as a viable course of action in an unpleasant, if not demeaning, situation for them as women. To move from being strategic actors towards social agency implies that women substance users first need to recognise why the 'object' of their choice is an addictive substance rather than some other 'object'.

Seeing pollution as a political issue
Rosaldo (1974, p. 38) has suggested that the 'ideas of purity and pollution, so often used to circumscribe female activities, may also be used as a basis for assertions of female solidarity, power or value'. In this specific context, Rosaldo was highlighting the fact that 'polluted' women who are feared, angry, or hold special or anomalous positions in society, 'take on powers uniquely their own'. In other words, these women are able to mobilise their own personal power, and indeed, further empower themselves by the very fact that they are seen to be 'polluted'.

While 'polluted' women are feared, they also have visible personal power and potential collective power. The social dynamics and beliefs surrounding the notion of pollution provide grounds for solidarity among women. Furthermore, extra-domestic ties with other women (e.g. women's self-help groups) are an important source of power and value in societies that create a firm division between the public and the private spheres (Rosaldo, 1974).

Here, I suggest that women substance users need to capitalise on their 'polluted' status and view pollution as a deeply political issue. In challenging traditional views of pollution, they gather strength. They expose how pollution is all about constructing moral judgements of what it means to be good, conforming women in society. This is a hidden, political process that is often used to divide women.

Publicising both pleasure and pain

Another challenge for women substance users is to see the potential for effective social action in de-privatising their pain. There exists a real need to make public women's experience of what I call patriarchal pain. This refers to any of a number of anguishing burdens women carry both publicly and privately in a gendered system of domination, and is the direct result of the countless contradictions inherent in women's social position.

Pleasure also needs to be made public rather than remain hidden. Women may use substances because they enjoy the pleasurable feeling. Substance use may be a diversion, if not an avoidance, of patriarchal pain as women struggle to comprehend masculinist reality and their female selves. There is a need for broader conceptions of substance use which move into the terrain of social structure and which uncover ideologies and practices surrounding women substance users. We need a vision of women as grounded in pleasure as well as pain. Acknowledging the differences of race, class, culture, age, sexual orientation and able bodiedness amongst women, there is a need to look at how women are able to struggle together to replace substance use, a form of pleasurable routine, with feminist affirming practices. We need to develop an acute, collective awareness of the energy of women's pleasure.

Conclusion

In conclusion, a basic contention of this chapter has been that developing a feminist perspective on, and response to, issues surrounding women and substance use is essential. Without a feminist awareness, there is a danger that the field of substance use will continue to remain politically sterile and insensitive to the needs of women sufferers.

This chapter has exposed quite clearly the need for social change, and the need for women substance users, researchers and clinicians to work towards this goal. Together, we need to demonstrate that the relations of patriarchy and women's use of substances go hand in hand. We need to be aware that the growth of inequalities and social divisions in societies produce greater problems surrounding the use of substances, specifically for women. In this light, we need to overturn traditional, oppressive ideologies on women substance users and help to bring these women out of an atmosphere of self-hatred, self-blame and fatalism. Women substance users hurt in our society. The level of social change demanded in this area needs to be deep enough to alleviate their pain.

Notes

1 At times, I use the words patriarchal and patriarchy in the text. These words refer to the gender ordering of society which is not only biased in favour of men, masculinity and male values, but also based primarily on male rather than female power structures and male rather than female based systems of social power distribution. My view is that a feminist analysis, in order to be comprehensive, should attempt to highlight inequalities in the gender, class and racial/ethnic ordering of society.
2 For a full discussion of feminist strategies in the field of substance use, see Ettorre (1992, pp. 137–144).

References

ALLAN, C. (1987) 'Seeking help for drinking problems from a community-based voluntary agency. Patterns of compliance amongst men and women', *British Journal of Addiction*, **82**, 1143–1147.

APPEL, C. (1990) 'Women, alcohol and society', paper presented to the 16th Annual Alcohol Epidemiology Symposium, Budapest, Hungary, 3–8 June, 1990.

BECKMAN, L. (1978) 'The self-esteem of women alcoholics', *Journal of Studies on Alcohol*, **39**(3), 491–498.

BEPKO, C. (Ed.) (1991) *Feminism and Addiction*, New York, The Haworth Press, Inc.

BOSTON WOMEN'S HEALTH COLLECTIVE (1978) PHILLIPS, A. and RAKUSEN, J. (Eds) *Our Bodies Ourselves: A Book By and For Women*, British Edition, Harmondsworth, Penguin.

BOVEY, S. (1989) *Being Fat is Not a Sin*, London, The Women's Press.

BRUUN, K., PAN, L. and REXED, I. (1975) *The Gentlemen's Club: International Control of Drugs and Alcohol*, Chicago, University of Chicago Press.

CHERNIN, K. (1981) *Womansize: The Tyranny of Slenderness*, London, The Women's Press.

CHERNIN, K. (1985) *The Hungry Self: Women, Eating and Identity*, London, Virago.

CURRAN, V. and GOLOMBOK, S. (1985) *Bottling it Up*, London, Faber and Faber.

DALY, M. (1984) *Pure Lust: Elemental Feminist Philosophy*, London, The Women's Press.

DAWN (1986) *Women and Stimulants*, London, Drugs, Alcohol and Women Nationally.

DOUGLAS, M. (1966) *Purity and Danger*, London, Routledge and Kegan Paul.

DOYAL, L. (1983) 'Women, health and the sexual division of labour: A case study of the Women's Health Movement in Britain', *International Journal of Health Services*, **13**(3), 373–387.

DOYAL, L. and ELSTON, M. (1986) 'Women, health and medicine', in BEECHEY, V. and WHITELEGG, E. (Eds) *Women in Britain Today*, Milton Keynes, Open University Press, pp. 173–209.

EHRENREICH, B. and ENGLISH, D. (1974) *Complaints and Disorders: The Sexual Politics of Sickness*, London, Compendium.

ERNST, S. and MAGUIRE, M. (1987) 'Introduction: living the question', in ERNST, S. and MAGUIRE, M. (Eds) *Living with the Sphinx*, London, The Women's Press.

ETTORRE, B. (1986) 'Women and drunken sociology: developing a feminist analysis', *Women's Studies International Forum*, 9(5), 515–520.

ETTORRE, B. (1989a) 'Women, substance abuse and self-help' in MACGREGOR, S. (Ed.) *Drugs and British Society*, London, Routledge.

ETTORRE, B. (1989b) 'Women and substance abuse: towards a feminist perspective or how to make dust fly', *Women's Studies International Forum*, 12(6), 593–602.

ETTORRE, E. (1992) *Women and Substance Use*, London, Macmillan and New Brunswick, New Jersey, Rutgers University Press.

ETTORRE, E. (forthcoming) 'Women and drug use with special reference to Finland: needing the "courage to see"' *Women's Studies International Forum*.

ETTORRE, E. and RISKA, E. (1992) 'Psychotropics, sociology and women: are the Halcyon days of the malestream over?' *Sociology of Health and Illness*, 15(4), 503–524.

FINCH, J. and GROVES, D. (1982) 'By women for women: caring for the frail elderly', *Women's Studies International Forum*, 5, 5.

FORTH-FINEGAN, J. L. (1991) 'Sugar and spice and everything nice: gender socialization and women's addiction — a literature review', in BEPKO, C. (Ed.) (1991) *Feminism and Addiction*, New York, The Haworth Press, Inc.

FRENCH, M. (1985) *Beyond Power: On Women, Men and Morals*, London, Sphere Books.

FRUCHTER, R. G., FATT, N., BOOTH, P. and LEIDEL, D. (1977) 'The women's health movement; Where are we now?' in DREIFUS, C. (Ed.) *Seizing our Bodies: The Politics of Women's Health*, New York, Vintage Books.

GARMARNIKOW, E., MORGAN, D., PURVIS, J. and TAYLORSON, D. (Eds) (1983) *The Public and the Private*, London, Heinneman.

GEFOU-MADIANOU, D. (Ed.) (1992) *Alcohol, Gender and Culture*, London and New York, Routledge.

GIDDENS, A. (1992) *The Transformation of Intimacy: Sexuality, Love and Eroticism in Modern Societies*, Cambridge, Polity Press.

GOSSOP, M. (1982) *Living with Drugs*, (First Edition), London, Temple Smith.

GRAHAM, H. (1983) 'Caring: a labour of love', in FINCH, J. and GROVES, D. (Eds) *A Labour of Love: Women, Work and Caring*, London, Routledge, pp. 13–30.

GRAHAM, H. (1987) 'Women's smoking and family health', *Social Science and Medicine*, 25(1), 47–56.

GRAHAM, H. (1990) 'Behaving well: women's health behaviour in context', in ROBERTS, H. (Ed.) *Women's Health Counts*, London, Routledge.

HAFNER, S. (1992) *Nice Girls Don't Drink*, New York, Bergin and Garvey.

HARPWOOD, D. (1982) *Tea and Tranquillisers*, London, Virago.

HIRSHMAN, J. and MUNTER, C. (1989) *Overcoming Overeating*, New York, Ballantine Books.

HOLLAND, J., RAMAZANOGLU, C. and SCOTT, S. (1990) 'AIDS. From panic stations to power relations: sociological perspectives and problems', *Sociology*, 24(3), 499–518.

HOLSTEIN, J. A. (1987) 'Producing gender effects on involuntary mental hospitalization', *Social Problems*, 34(2), 141–155.

JACOBSON, B. (1981) *The Ladykillers: Why Smoking is a Feminist Issue*, London, Pluto Press.

JACOBSON, B. (1986) *Beating the Ladykillers: Women and Smoking*, London, Pluto Press.

KALANT, O. J. (1980) 'Sex differences in alcohol and drug problems: some highlights', in KALANT, O. J. (Ed.) *Alcohol and Drug Problems in Women*, London, Pluto Press.

KITZINGER, C. (1991) Feminism, psychology and the paradox of power, *Feminism and Psychology: An International Journal*, 1(1).

KRAMARAE, C. and TREICHLER, P. A. (1985) *A Feminist Dictionary*, London, Pandora Press.

LAWRENCE, M. (Ed.) (1987) *Fed Up and Hungry: Women, Oppression and Food*, London, The Women's Press.

LEWIN, E. (1987) 'By design: reproductive strategies and the meaning of motherhood', in HOMANS, H. (Ed.) *The sexual politics of reproduction*, Aldershot, Gower.

MACGREGOR, S. and ETTORRE, B. (1987) 'From treatment to rehabilitation — aspects of the evolution of British policy on care of drug-takers', in DORN, N. and SOUTH, N. (Eds) *Land fit for Heroin?* London, Macmillan, pp. 125-145.

MASON, M. (1991) 'Woman and shame: kin and culture', in BEPKO, C. (Ed.) (1991) *Feminism and Addiction*, New York, The Haworth Press, Inc.

MCCONVILLE, B. (1983) *Women Under the Influence: Alcohol and Its Impact*, London, Virago.

MELVILLE, J. (1984) *The Tranquilliser Trap and How to Get Out of it*, London, Fontana Paperbacks.

MILLER, D. (1991) 'Are we keeping up with Oprah? A treatment and training model for addictions and interpersonal violence', in BEPKO, C. (Ed.) (1991) *Feminism and Addiction*, New York, The Haworth Press, Inc.

ORBACH, S. (1978) *Fat is a Feminist Issue*, London, Hamlyn Publications.

ORBACH, S. (1986) *Hunger Strike*, London, Faber and Faber.

PERRY, L. (1979) *Women and Drug Use: An Unfeminine Dependency*, London, Institute for the Study of Drug Dependency.

RAYMOND, J. (1986) *A Passion for Friends: Towards a Philosophy of Female Affection*, London, The Women's Press.

ROSALDO, M. Z. (1974) 'Woman, Culture and Society: A Theoretical Overview', in ROSALDO, M. Z. and LAMPHERE, L. (Eds) *Woman, Culture and Society*, Stanford California, Stanford University Press, pp. 17-42.

ROSE, H. (1986) 'Beyond Masculinist Realities: A Feminist Epistemology for the Sciences', in BLEIER, R. (Ed.) *Feminist Approaches to Science*, Oxford, Pergamon Press, pp. 57-76.

ROSENBAUM, M. (1981) *Women on Heroin*, New Brunswick, New Jersey, Rutgers University Press.

RUZEK, S. (1978) *The Women's Health Movement: Feminist Alternatives to Medical Control*, New York, Praeger.

SARGENT, M. (1992) *Women, Drugs and Policy in Sydney, London and Amsterdam*, Aldershot, Avebury.

STEINEM, G. (1979) 'These are not the Best Years of Your Life', *Ms*, 8(3), 64-68.

THOM, B. (1984) 'A process approach to women's use of alcohol services', *British Journal of Addiction*, 79(4), 377-382.

THOM, B. (1986) 'Sex differences in help-seeking for alcohol problems-1. The barriers to help-seeking', *British Journal of Addiction*, 81(6), 777-788.

THOM, B. (1987) 'Sex differences in help-seeking for alcohol problems-2. Entry into treatment', *British Journal of Addiction*, 82(9), 989-997.

THUNHURST, C. (1982) *It Makes You Sick: The Politics of the NHS*, London, Pluto Press.

VANCE, C. (1984) 'Pleasure and danger: toward a politics of sexuality', in VANCE, C. (Ed.) *Pleasure and Danger: Exploring Female Sexuality*, London, Routledge and Kegan Paul.

VAN NIEUWKERK, K. (1992) 'Female entertainers in Egypt: drinking and gender roles', in GEFOU-MADIANOU, D. (Ed.) *Alcohol, Gender and Culture*, London and New York, Routledge.

WOLFSON, D. and MURRAY, J. (Eds) (1986) *Women and Dependency: Women's Personal Accounts of Drug and Alcohol Problems*, London, DAWN.

Chapter 7

Surviving by Smoking

Hilary Graham

In contrast to other areas of women's health, there is an absence of feminist research and feminist debate about cigarette smoking. There is only a handful of studies which seek to understand women's smoking behaviour in the context of the social divisions which shape their identities and their daily lives. The lack of a feminist agenda around women's smoking would be unimportant if cigarette smoking was not related either to women's health or to gender divisions in any significant way. But cigarette smoking is connected to both, and in increasingly pronounced ways. Cigarette smoking is currently identified as the major single cause of disease and premature mortality in industrialized capitalist countries, and is increasingly implicated as a cause of women's mortality and of ill-health and death in children. Further, smoking patterns are changing in ways which are tying cigarette smoking more closely to gender divisions and to other hierarchies of oppression. In Britain, as in other capitalist countries, cigarette smoking is emerging as a habit acquired and sustained by those who occupy disadvantaged positions within the social hierarchy.

This chapter explores some of the connections between cigarette smoking and social divisions. Drawing on the mainstream quantitative data on women's smoking and the more limited tradition of qualitative research, the chapter seeks to develop a perspective sensitive to the ways in which women experience and resist oppression in their daily lives. The chapter begins by briefly summarising the epidemiological evidence on the health risks of smoking before turning to review the changing patterns and contexts of women's smoking in Britain. The second part of the chapter looks more directly at women's experiences of smoking. It focuses on White[1] women caring for children in low-income households. Their accounts suggest that smoking is one of the ways women handle and defuse the contradictory pressures that structure their daily lives. It provides a way of keeping going when women have little going for them. The habit identified as the major cause of premature death and childhood ill-health in Britain is — paradoxically — one which many women identify as essential to their survival and to the survival of their families.

As in other areas of health research, the chapter relies on data which provide a problematic base on which to build feminist understandings of women's experiences. As an introduction to the central parts of the chapter, the section below briefly highlights some of the problems.

Researching Women's Smoking: Some Problems with the Data

There are four characteristics of research on smoking in Britain which pose problems for the development of feminist perspectives on women's smoking.

First, most of what is known about women's smoking derives from quantitative surveys which measure women's smoking status but do not record the everyday experiences which sustain their smoking behaviour. In contrast to other areas of women's health where there is now a rich seam of qualitative research (e.g. pregnancy and motherhood: see Oakley, 1979; Wiles, this volume), there are only a few studies of women's smoking in which analyses stay close to the understandings that women have of themselves and their lives. Smoking research is still very much a field in which statistics speak louder than words. The second part of the chapter draws on these analyses. Women's accounts are woven into the text, providing a separate but linked commentary on the place of smoking in their lives.

Second, the changing patterns of smoking are mapped from the answers people give researchers about their smoking status and their cigarette consumption. A comparison of self-reported data with tax data and other information derived from the sale of tobacco products suggests that these answers underestimate both prevalence and consumption (Todd, 1978; Jackson and Benglehole, 1985). There are likely to be gender-specific factors which work against disclosure of cigarette smoking among women, including the cultural sanctions operating against smoking among some women in South Asian communities, and against smoking in pregnancy and motherhood among all women.

Third, smoking surveys rely on measures of social position which distort and obscure the dimensions of women's identity which feminist research has sought to make visible. For example, feminist researchers seeking to trace the links between women's smoking and women's lives are forced to rely on measures which accord a privileged status to marriage and cohabiting relationships with men. Thus, women are defined as either living alone (as a single, separated, divorced or widowed woman) or as living with a male partner (as a married or cohabiting woman). Cohabitation is defined in heterosexual terms and women's domestic and sexual relationships with women are written out of the classification. There is, therefore, nothing to be learned from the volume of smoking research about how the domestic lives of women living with women, in sexual and non-sexual relationships, affect their smoking behaviour. There is nothing to be learned either on the broader questions of how sexuality is linked to smoking status, and whether the smoking careers and identities of lesbians are different from the careers and identities of straight women. The little information available derives from small-scale studies (Buenting, 1993).

Information on the class background of women smokers again derives from a classification procedure in which women's position is mediated by their relationship with men. Women who are married to, or living with, men are ascribed a class position on the basis of their partners' current or last occupation. Women living alone, like women in a cohabitating relationship with another woman, earn their class position directly on the basis of their own occupation. These different classification procedures mean that links between women's occupation and their smoking status are obscured (Graham and Hunt, 1994).

The measures that tap the ethnic identity of women smokers are similarly problematic. Until the 1980s, surveys relied on women's country of birth as a measure of ethnic identity. More recent one-off surveys rely on classifications based on ethnic identity, using a range of different classifications (Cox, 1987; Oakley *et al.*, 1992). None of the continuous surveys of smoking behaviour publish information on the ethnic identity of smokers.

A final caveat needs to be entered about the data on women's smoking. A major source of information on smoking status, the General Household Survey, refers to cigarette smoking. While very few women use other forms of tobacco, a small minority of men smoke pipes and cigars. Excluding these forms of tobacco-use has the effect of making the decline in male smoking prevalence more pronounced, and the gap in the smoking prevalence rates of women and men narrower than it would otherwise be. Recording cigarette smoking only also has the effect of exaggerating gender differences in smoking cessation (Jarvis, 1984; Jarvis and Johnson, 1988).

These four features of smoking surveys raise questions about what can be gleaned from a quantitative research tradition which obscures women's experiences and masks key dimensions of their identity and social position. However, this tradition provides the only available source of insight to date into the links between women's smoking and women's lives.

Cigarette Smoking and the Nation's Health

Cigarette smoking is regarded as the single most important cause of disease and premature death in Britain. It is estimated that just under 20 per cent of all deaths in developed countries are attributable to cigarette smoking (Peto *et al.* 1992). In addition to its links with coronary heart disease, smoking has been identified as the primary cause of lung cancer, accounting for 80 per cent of lung cancer deaths in Britain (Secretary of State, 1992).

Increasing attention has been paid to the health effects of women's smoking (Chollat-Traquet, 1992). While lung cancer mortality among men in Britain has been declining since the 1970s, it is still rising among women. In Scotland, female deaths from lung cancer have exceeded those from breast cancer since 1984, and in certain areas of northern England, lung cancer has recently overtaken breast cancer as the main cause of female cancer death (CRC, 1992). In addition to the damage to women's health, epidemiological research and health promotion policy have highlighted the dangers that women's smoking represents for children (Royal College of Physicians, 1992; Secretary of State, 1992). Maternal smoking during pregnancy and infancy is seen as a major risk factor for childhood morbidity and mortality. It has been linked to a greater risk of miscarriage and of death during the latter stages of pregnancy and the first week of life. It is also linked to low birth-weight, to sudden infant death syndrome and to a range of health problems affecting the physical growth and educational development of young children (Gillies and Wakefield, 1993).

Such evidence on the risks of smoking has been incorporated into perspectives which emphasise that it is lifestyles rather than living conditions that shape people's health (Townsend, *et al.*, 1988). These perspectives lend support to government policies which seek to change what people do rather than the circumstances in which they live. A long-running theme in British social policy, the lifestyle emphasis is now inscribed into the objectives of health policy. The government has set targets for England for the year 2000, which lay down the scale of reduction to be achieved in cigarette smoking and in other injurious habits, including the consumption of alcohol and saturated fatty acids (Secretary of State, 1992). The meeting of these lifestyle targets is seen to provide the means by which reductions in the major causes of mortality, like lung cancer and coronary heart disease, can be secured. Tackling the material factors associated with poor health and health-damaging behaviours is not part of the government's health agenda. No parallel targets have been set for improvements in the circumstances in which people experience poor health and find it hard to adopt health-promoting lifestyles.

While health policy plays down the significance of social and material circumstances, the evidence on women's smoking suggests that they are integral to the maintenance of smoking habits. They provide the contexts in which and against which women continue to smoke.

The Changing Patterns of Women's Smoking in Britain

Increasing public awareness of the health risks of smoking has been associated with a decline in cigarette smoking in Britain. However, smoking prevalence has not fallen uniformly across the population. Instead, it has declined in ways that have profoundly altered the social distribution of cigarette smoking. Across the last four decades, its gender and class profile has been transformed; the limited evidence on ethnic identity suggests that smoking among women has remained predominantly a habit of White women. The new social distribution of cigarette smoking has emerged across a period in which social and economic changes have widened inequalities in living standards and life chances in Britain. This section looks in turn at the changing gender and class patterns of smoking, and at the economic contexts in which these changes have occurred.

The Changing Gender Profile of Cigarette Smoking

Seventy years ago, smoking had a clear male identity. Tobacco consumption among women had only just reached recordable levels

(Figure 7.1). The new female smokers were smoking manufactured cigarettes; the traditional forms of consumption, like pipes, cigars, snuff and tobacco for chewing, remained male habits (Wald *et al.*, 1988). Through the 1920s and 1930s, female tobacco consumption increased steadily with a particularly sharp rise during the war years of 1939 to 1945. The war-time increase was linked to a rapid fall in the age at which women took up smoking. By 1945, one in three women aged twenty was a smoker. As with men, regular smoking had become firmly established as a habit acquired during adolescence and early adulthood (McKennell and Thomas, 1967). The trends in women's and men's cigarette smoking in the post-war period are mapped out in Figure 7.2. It suggests that smoking prevalence started to decline earlier and more rapidly among men than women. The exclusion of cigar and pipe smoking exaggerates this gender difference. Nonetheless, it is clear that men have found it easier to turn away from cigarette smoking than women. The proportion of adults who have never smoked cigarettes has risen much more rapidly among men than among women. The proportion of ex-cigarette smokers has also increased more rapidly among men than women (Wald *et al.*, 1988; OPCS, 1992).

The result of these gender differences in acquisition and cessation is a shift in the gender profile of cigarette smoking. This shift is most pronounced among young people. Here, what was once an exclusively male activity is now a habit more strongly associated with being a woman. Regular smoking among 11 to 15-year-olds in Britain is now more common among girls than boys (Lader and Matheson, 1991). Among those aged 16 to 24, too, smoking prevalence rates are now higher for women than men (OPCS, 1992).

Smoking among young women is a habit acquired by White women. Among White women, higher rates of cigarette smoking are reported among women born in Ireland than among UK-born women. Rates are also higher among women living in Northern Ireland, Wales and Scotland than among women in England (Barker *et al.*, 1989; OPCS 1992). Reported rates of smoking among young Asian and African-Caribbean women are low, although there is some evidence which points to an increase in smoking prevalence among young African-Caribbean women (Oakley *et al.*, 1992). These patterns are repeated in adulthood. In the national Health and Lifestyle Survey, conducted in the mid-1980s, one in five African-Caribbean women and one in twenty South Asian women reported that they were cigarette smokers. One in three White women stated that they were smokers (Cox 1987; Graham, unpublished data).

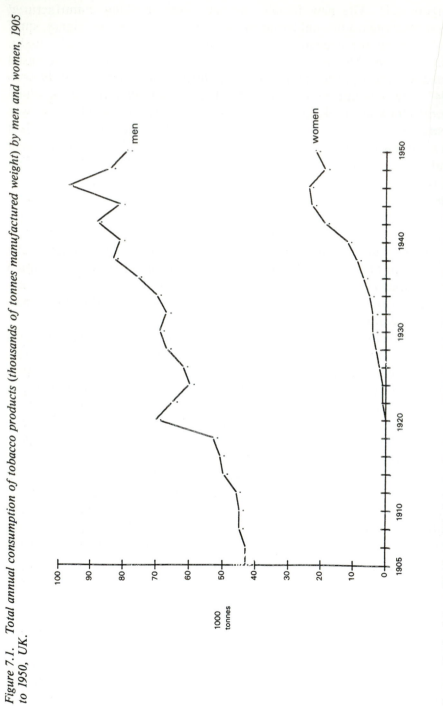

Figure 7.1. Total annual consumption of tobacco products (thousands of tonnes manufactured weight) by men and women, 1905 to 1950, UK.

Source: Derived from Wald, N., Kiryluk, S., Darby, S., Doll, R., Pike, M. and Peto, R. (1988) *UK Smoking Statistics*, Table 1.3.

Figure 7.2. Prevalence of cigarette smoking among men and women aged 16 and over, 1948 to 1990, Britain.

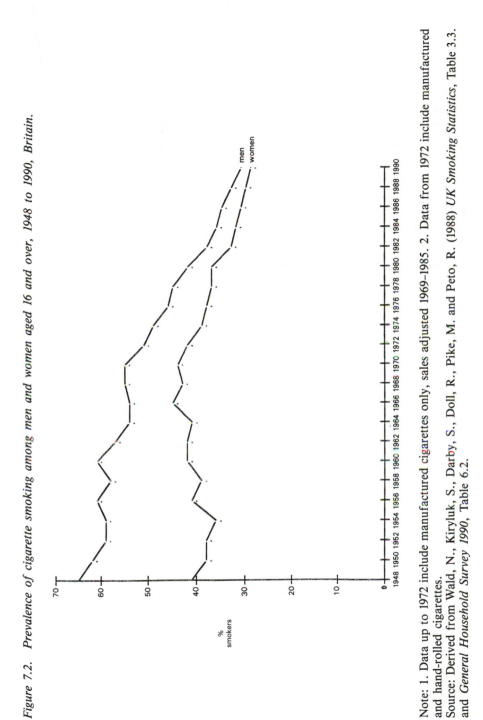

Note: 1. Data up to 1972 include manufactured cigarettes only, sales adjusted 1969–1985. 2. Data from 1972 include manufactured and hand-rolled cigarettes.
Source: Derived from Wald, N., Kiryluk, S., Darby, S., Doll, R., Pike, M. and Peto, R. (1988) *UK Smoking Statistics*, Table 3.3. and *General Household Survey 1990*, Table 6.2.

The Changing Class Profile of Cigarette Smoking

It is not only the gender identity of cigarette smoking which has altered radically across the last four decades. There has also been a rapid shift in its class base. There is little evidence on the class background of female smokers in the early decades of the century. The limited information suggests that cigarette smoking was a symbol of emancipation and sexual equality, a fashion accessory for affluent, upwardly-mobile city-living women (Ernster, 1985; Jacobson, 1986). In the 1940s and early 1950s, the proportion of women who smoked was higher among those in higher-income households and significantly lower among women living with unemployed male partners (Wald *et al.*, 1988). By the 1950s, cigarette smoking displayed a uniform class distribution: just over 40 per cent of women in all social classes reported that they smoked cigarettes (Figure 7.3).

Figure 7.3.   Prevalence of cigarette smoking among women by social class, 1958, Britain.

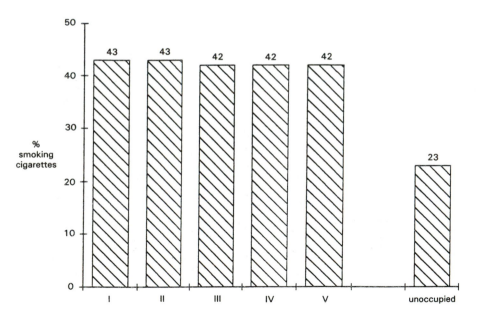

Notes: 1. Married women are classified on the basis of their husband's occupation. 2. Those who are retired and who have been unemployed for less than two months are classified according to their previous occupation. 3. Those who have been unemployed for more than two months are classified as unoccupied.
Source: Derived from Wald, N., Kiryluk, S., Darby, S., Doll, R., Pike, M. and Peto, R. (1988) *UK Smoking Statistics*, Table 5.5.

Since the 1960s, a sharp class gradient has emerged in cigarette smoking among women and men. Data from the General Household Survey point to a prevalence rate that is more than twice as high among women in households with an unskilled manual head of household (36 per cent) than among women in the highest socio-economic group of professional groups (16 per cent) (Figure 7.4).

The emergence of this pronounced class gradient does not reflect class differences in health knowledge. The majority of women in all socio-economic groups recognise the health risks of smoking (Marsh and Matheson, 1983; Ben-Shlomo *et al.*, 1991). The emergence of a class gradient reflects class differences in the extent to which women have put their health knowledge into practice. Women in higher socio-economic groups have changed their smoking behaviour in line with health education advice earlier and in larger numbers than women in poorer socio-economic circumstances. As a result, sharp class differences have

Figure 7.4.   Prevalence of cigarette smoking among women by socio-economic group, Britain, 1990.

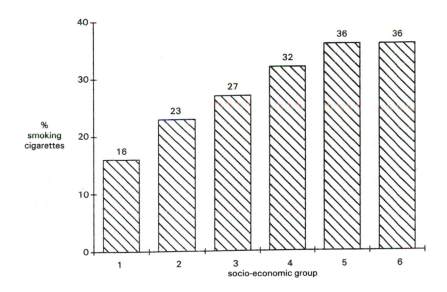

Key: 1 = Professional, 2 = Employers, 3 = Intermediate & junior non-manual, 4 = Skilled manual, 5 = Semi-skilled manual, 6 = Unskilled manual.
Notes: Married and cohabiting women whose male partners are in the household are classified according to their partner's present (or last) job.
Source: Derived from OPCS *General Household Survey 1990*, Table 6.4.

Figure 7.5. Smoking prevalence among expectant mothers before pregnancy by social class, 1990, UK.

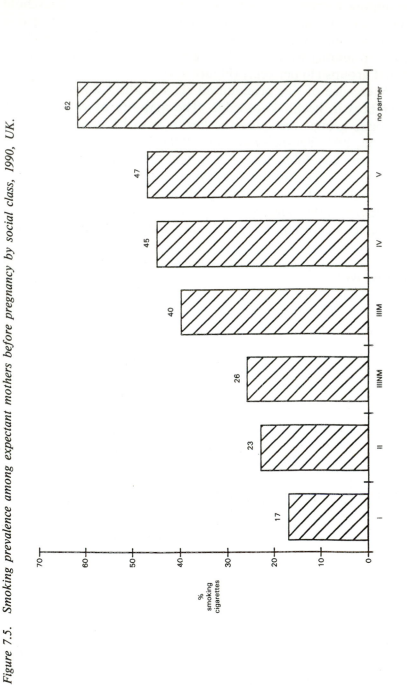

Notes: Social class defined by current or last occupation of husband/male partner. Those without a male partner are classified separately.
Source: White, A., Freeth, S. and O'Brien, M. (1992) *Infant Feeding 1990*, Table 2.11.

Figure 7.6. Smoking cessation among expectant mothers by social class, 1990, UK.

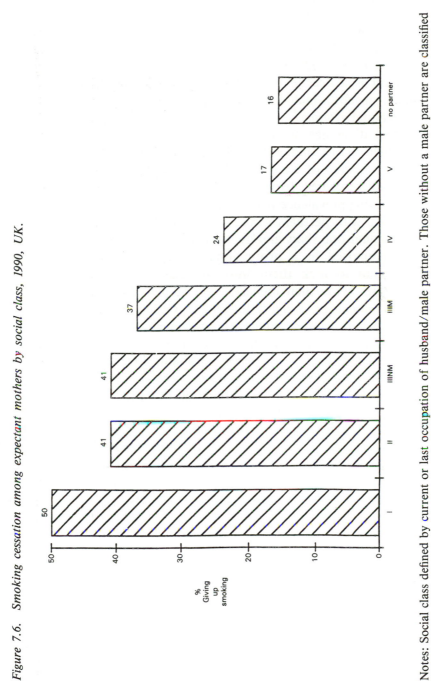

Notes: Social class defined by current or last occupation of husband/male partner. Those without a male partner are classified separately.

Source: White, A., Freeth, S. and O'Brien, M. (1992) *Infant Feeding 1990*, Table 2.11.

emerged in smoking acquisition and smoking cessation. For every hundred women who are current smokers in professional households, there are 388 women who have never smoked and 138 ex-smokers. For every hundred women in unskilled manual households who are current smokers, there are 125 women who have never smoked and fifty-three ex-smokers (OPCS, 1992). The result of these differences in acquisition and cessation is a decline in smoking prevalence among women in professional groups which has yet to be repeated among women in unskilled manual groups.

The class differences in women's smoking are particularly marked among women before and during pregnancy. Figure 7.5, based on a 1990 national survey of expectant mothers, confirms the steep class gradient among women living with male partners. In this group, reported smoking prevalence prior to pregnancy was three times higher among women with partners whose current or last occupation was an unskilled manual one than among women with partners currently or previously employed in a professional occupation. Among women without a man to lock them into the class classification system, prevalence rates are at their highest. Over 60 per cent of lone mothers begin their pregnancies as cigarette smokers (White *et al.*, 1992).

Most pregnant women enter their pregnancies aware of the health risks of smoking for themselves, their unborn baby and other children in the household (Madley *et al.*, 1989; Graham, 1993a). A significant minority — between 25 per cent and 30 per cent — give up smoking in pregnancy, particularly in the first three months (Gillies and Wakefield, 1993). But the women who quit are disproportionately those living in the more advantaged socio-economic circumstances. Women who live in the poorest socio-economic circumstances, as lone mothers and women living with male partners in social class V, face greater barriers in changing their smoking status. As Figure 7.6 records, smoking cessation rates in pregnancy are a mirror image of smoking prevalence rates prior to pregnancy: it is lone mothers and women living with men in social class V who are least likely to become ex-smokers.

Widening Inequalities in Income

The new social distribution of cigarette smoking has emerged across a period marked by social and economic change. It is not only the lifestyles but the living conditions of the population which have altered since the 1950s. The emergence of a class gradient in women's smoking has coincided with a widening of inequalities in income and living standard between households at the top and the bottom of the income distribution. Since the 1950s, households on higher incomes have been getting richer relative to households on lower incomes (Wilkinson, 1989; House of Commons, 1991). In other words, cigarette smoking has become increasingly associated with socio-economic disadvantage at a time when more men and women are living in disadvantaged circumstances.

Households with children have been particularly affected by widening income inequalities and are increasingly likely to find themselves trying to survive on a low income. In 1979, one child in ten was growing up in a household with an income below 50 per cent of average income, a threshold taken as an unofficial poverty line in national and international surveys. In 1991, the proportion was one in three (Department of Social Security, 1993). The increasing risks of poverty among families have not been borne equally by all households with children. It has fallen particularly on lone mothers. As the number of lone mother households has increased across the 1970s, 1980s and 1990s, their financial circumstances have deteriorated. In the early 1970s, a third of lone mothers received supplementary benefit, the precursor of income support. By the early 1990s, the proportion had doubled. Over 70 per cent of lone mothers are dependent on the minimum levels of income provided by income support (Burghes, 1993). The evidence suggests that these minimum levels are insufficient to meet the basic and essential needs of children and their parents. The income support of a lone mother with two children would need to be 26 per cent higher (£23.08 a week at 1993 prices) if it was to meet the basic costs of bringing up a family (Oldfield and Yu, 1993).

These changes in the economic welfare of households provide an important backdrop to the trends in women's smoking. They suggest that cigarette smoking among women has become increasingly associated with poor socio-economic circumstances at a time when more women are caring for children on low incomes and on benefit. Specifically, it has become associated with being a lone mother across a period in which the number of lone mothers has increased sharply and their financial circumstances have worsened. The section below examines these connections between smoking and caring on a low income.

Smoking and Caring on a Low Income

The changing patterns of cigarette smoking in Britain suggest that those in more privileged positions in the gender and class hierarchies have found it easier to adopt and maintain a non-smoking identity. Conversely, there appear to be experiences which, along with gender and class disadvantage, make it harder to be a non-smoker. The lives of women caring in low-income households shed light on the experiences which connect gender and class to smoking behaviour. Reflecting the ethnic differences in cigarette smoking, it is White women's experiences which resource this section. It draws on women's accounts that have been previously published as well as unpublished data from interviews conducted as part of a survey of the everyday lives of mothers caring for pre-school children (Graham, 1985).

The section looks in turn at the links between smoking and gender responsibilities, and smoking and class circumstances. While these two dimensions are experienced together, separating them illuminates the complex ways in which smoking is enmeshed in women's lives.

Smoking and Gender Responsibilities

Family life in Britain is sustained by a gendered division of labour in which women take primary responsibility for childcare and domestic labour (Kiernan, 1992). In households with pre-school children, most mothers work full-time on their caring and domestic responsibilities. In these households, the gendered division of labour is at its sharpest (Pahl, 1984). The combined responsibilities of childcare and domestic labour make for long working days — and often long working nights. It is work structured by the timetable of other people's needs, with the shopping and cooking, washing and ironing, cleaning and clearing away fitted around the routines of caring for children and partners' hours of work.

> You're on the go from seven in the morning and you're on call more or less all night, every night, whereas you're not when you're working. Your boss isn't going to ring you up at eleven o'clock at night and say come and take a letter, whereas if the baby cries, you can't say I've finished for the day, tough luck (Unnamed mother in Oakley, 1979, p. 39).

> I think looking after children is the hardest job going and the one where you get the least preparation and training for. To be

quite honest, that's how I feel. Very, very demanding in time, energy, affection and it's not a job you've got from nine in the morning till five at night. It's 24 hours a day, especially as my son has only just started going through the night and he's four and a half. Very demanding on all fronts. Demanding 24 hours of attention is a bit much and I think you need — well I need — a time without them to regain a little bit of sanity (Unnamed mother, in Graham, 1985).

Where women have spoken of their caring experiences, they have noted how they try to weave other and more self-directed routines into the schedule of childcare and housework. These breaks from caring, principally of the coffee and tea variety, have both a symbolic and a material significance, marking out adult time in which mothers can rest and 'refuel'. For smokers, cigarettes appear to play a central part in this process of making and marking out time for oneself: anticipated breaks when domestic responsibilities can be temporarily put to one side and the mother can enter a social world which is not exclusively focused on childcare.

I smoke when I'm sitting down, having a cup of coffee. It's part and parcel of resting. Definitely, because it doesn't bother me if I haven't got a cigarette when I'm working. If I can keep working, doing the housework and the washing and the ironing and things like that, and I'm busy, I won't bother but if I'm sitting down chatting or sitting having a cup of coffee, then I smoke. If I'm busy, it doesn't bother me, but it's nice to sit down afterwards and have a cigarette (Unnamed mother quoted in Graham, 1993b, p. 182).

Smoking is time for myself. In the morning I have a cigarette, but I wait till I'm back from taking Sue to school, then I can sit down with a cup of tea and spend a little time sorting myself out for the day (Unnamed mother quoted in Nicotinell, 1993, p. 32).

After Julie is in bed, we'll sit down as often as not and watch telly and I'll smoke a cigarette. I always have, even when I was working. It's my way of saying, 'that's it. I've done my work for today' (Unnamed mother quoted in Graham, 1976, p. 403).

Providing a way of structuring time and containing their domestic responsibilities, mothers have described how cigarette smoking is used to control their mood. It provides a way of relieving the boredom and isolation that can go with full-time caring on a low income.

> I smoke less when I'm not with others, a lot of it's out of boredom. I don't go out much, about once a fortnight, so I'm here on my own every night once the baby's in bed.

> I'm a heavier smoker because I'm in all day. I don't go out, don't drink and don't have a car. It's the only pleasure I have.

> I think it's because I'm bored, I smoke. I have no one else to talk to. I don't go out in the evenings. I feel a lot better when I'm busy. I don't have a lot of friends around here (Unnamed mothers quoted in Wells, 1987, p. 11).

Recent studies have pointed to one particularly crucial aspect of the mood-management functions of smoking for women with young children. They have noted how smoking is experienced as a way of coping with stress and anger: a way of re-imposing order and calm when mothers feel their energy and patience is giving way (Graham, 1976, 1987; Wells, 1987).

When faced with demands they cannot meet, mothers have described how they create a space — symbolic if not real — between them and their children and fill this space with a self-directed activity. Smoking a cigarette provides a self-directed activity which can be accessed instantly when mothers feel that their breaking point has been reached (Graham, 1987, 1988). A recent survey of mothers with children under the age of seven underlined how central cigarette smoking can be to the management of anger and the avoidance of physical abuse. Over 70 per cent of the smokers felt that smoking helped them to calm down when they felt like shouting at their children, and over 50 per cent reported that smoking helped them to calm down when they felt like smacking their children (Nicotinell, 1993). Such evidence points to the contradictory pressures bearing on women caring for children. The habit identified as one of the most important risk factors in childhood morbidity and mortality is experienced as a preventive strategy for non-accidental injury. In other words, maternal smoking is a habit through which the welfare of children is simultaneously threatened and protected.

> I send them up to their bedroom when they're getting too much for me. When I see the danger signs looming, I think they're best out of the way. I sit down and have a cigarette and a cup of tea. After 10 minutes, I feel guilty and call them down. Usually the crisis has passed by then (Unnamed mother, unpublished data from Graham, 1985).

[I'm very likely to smoke] when I'm making the tea. The two older ones come home from school, the baby's hungry and all four of them are hungry. They are all fighting and screaming in here and the dinner's cooking in the kitchen. I'm ready to blow up so I light up a cigarette. It calms me down when I'm under so much stress. Since the baby was born, you feel at the end of your tether and a cigarette makes me feel better, helps me cope. I feel it's better than throwing him about and tearing my hair out.

I enjoy a cigarette. My friends all smoke and I get a bit irritable if I give up for any length of time. It acts as a safety valve for me really (Unnamed mothers quoted in Graham, 1993a, p. 58 and p. 62).

Smoking and Material Circumstances

Parents bringing up children on low incomes spend more of the little they have on collective necessities, like food and fuel, than do better-off households. They spend less, both in absolute and relative terms, on personal items, like clothes and shoes, where purchases, however essential, can be deferred. It is a strategy for survival which leaves a mother constantly aware of her family's poverty: of what they have not got and what they can not do. It is a lifestyle of enforced exclusion from the communities to which they belong.

I'm a member of the Church Council and a governor of the [primary] School, those things I've kept up. I was on the PTA at St. Joseph's [secondary school], I've dropped that. I did get to the point where I had no clothes to wear to go . . . How could I go to those meetings with trainers with no soles and jeans with holes in? . . . I felt I could go to the primary school like that and they would understand, but not the secondary school, because the children are that much older. I don't think they would want me to turn up looking like that and I certainly wouldn't want to inflict it on them (Unnamed mother quoted in Cohen, 1991, p. 5).

These budgeting strategies would suggest that spending on tobacco, as a non-essential personal item, would be low. However, low-income households spend *more* on tobacco than households on higher incomes. Like food and fuel, spending on tobacco is inversely related to income: more is spent proportionately on tobacco as household income falls.

More is also spent in absolute terms in lower-income households: it is the one item of expenditure where the poor spend more than the rich. While many would regard it a luxury item, tobacco spending has the hallmark of a necessity. It is something that mothers identify as essential to their survival.

> I try to cut down to save money but cigarettes are my one luxury and at the moment they feel a bit like a necessity (Unnamed mother quoted in Graham, 1988, p. 375).

> I couldn't face a day without cigarettes. That's all we've got now (Unnamed mother quoted in Simms and Smith, 1986, p. 78).

Mothers' accounts suggest smoking provides a way of getting through hours, days and weeks of cutting back. Cigarette smoking provides a time-out from the grind of cutting back and making do. Male partners are seen to have other and more real forms of escape: for women, however, cigarettes may provide the only moment when the struggle for financial survival can be suspended and they can join a world of personal consumption that most adults take for granted.

> My husband goes out three times a week drinking with his mates. I don't go. Smoking is my form of relaxation.

> My boyfriend has his pleasure. He drinks. The only pleasure I have is smoking (Unnamed mothers quoted in Simms and Smith, 1986, pp. 78–9).

Smoking can provide a particularly important resource during the times of crises that puncture the lives of those struggling against material disadvantage. Smoking is a means of survival, a way of keeping oneself and one's family together through redundancy and long-term illness, and during the threat of eviction and the reality of homelessness (Oakley, 1989; Graham, 1993b).

> I was going to go on valium, but in the end I thought no, don't and I coped, I coped without it. I was afraid that if I started anything that I wouldn't be able to give up or get off it, so I went to cigarettes, and that was something I couldn't give up ... When I'm alright I don't smoke, but when I'm under stress, I do.

> How much are you smoking now? (Interviewer)

> Twenty now, I'm cutting them down, but I smoke because everything I have wanted has been ruined. I haven't got anything else left now. (Pregnant lone mother with a two-year

old daughter; living in a women's refuge having left a violent marriage. Quoted in Oakley, 1989, p. 321).

Conclusions

The patterns of cigarette smoking are changing in Britain in ways that are tying the habit more closely to the experience of disadvantage and oppression. Similar trends are evident in other capitalist countries (Pierce, 1989; Chollat-Traquet, 1992). Drawing on British data, the chapter has sought to develop a feminist perspective on these trends in smoking behaviour, highlighting how cigarette smoking is enmeshed in the strategies by which women experience and survive inequality.

This chapter has focused particularly on the experience of gender and class inequality, as the contexts in which smoking careers in Britain are established and sustained. In focusing on the connections between gender and class, other dimensions of identity and oppression, including 'race', sexuality and disability, have inevitably been placed in shadow. However, the themes which emerge may have a significance beyond the lives of women for whom gender and class divisions represent the major axes of oppression in their daily lives. The themes suggest that smoking, identified as the major cause of premature death in Britain, is a way of getting through everyday life. Specifically, smoking is a way of living with and living through the experiences that go with social inequality. In the context of gender and class oppression, it provides a resource which can be accessed instantly when caring responsibilities are many and material resources are few.

The evidence suggests that women recognise the contradictory kind of support that smoking provides. They are aware that the habit which sustains them and supports the welfare of their children is also damaging to their health and the health of their children. Cigarette smoking thus illuminates, in a particularly sharp way, the toll that social divisions take on the welfare of women and their children.

Note

1 'Black' is often introduced with a capital letter to signify that it is a political category, forged out of social inequalities and not out of biological differences. 'White' has been capitalised in the same way, to indicate that the position and experiences of White as well as Black people in Britain are socially constructed and not biologically determined.

References

BARKER, M. E., McCLEAN, S. I., McKENNA, P. G., REID, N. G., STRAIN, J. J., THOMPSON, K. A., WILLIAMSON, A. P. and WRIGHT, M. E. (1989) *Diet, Lifestyle and Health in Northern Ireland*, Centre for Applied Health Studies, Coleraine, University of Ulster.

BEN-SHLOMO, B., SHEIHAM, A. and MARMOT, M. (1991) 'Smoking and health' in JOWELL, R., BROOK, L. and TAYLOR, B. (eds) *British Social Attitudes: the 8th Report*, Aldershot, Dartmouth.

BUENTING, J. A. (1993) 'Health life-styles of lesbian and heterosexual women', in NOERAGER STERN, P. (Ed.) *Lesbian Health: What Are The Issues?* London, Taylor and Francis.

BLAXTER, M. (1990) *Health and Lifestyles*, London, Routledge.

BURGHES, L. (1993) *One Parent Families: Policy Options for the 1990s*, York, Family Policy Studies Centre/Joseph Rowntree Foundation.

CANCER RESEARCH CAMPAIGN (CRC) (1992) *Facts on Cancer*, London, CRC.

CHOLLAT-TRAQUET, C. (1992) *Women and Tobacco*, Geneva, WHO.

COHEN, R. (1991) *Just About Surviving, Life on Income Support: Quality of Life and the Impact of Local Services*, London, Family Service Units.

COX, B. D. (Ed.) (1987) *Health and Lifestyle Survey*, London, Health Promotion Research Trust.

DEPARTMENT OF SOCIAL SECURITY (1993) *Social Security Statistics 1993*, London, HMSO.

ERNSTER, V. (1985) 'Mixed messages for women; a social history of cigarette smoking and advertising', *New York State Journal of Medicine*, July, 335–40.

GILLIES, P. A. and WAKEFIELD, M. (1993) 'Smoking in pregnancy', *Current Obstetrics and Gynaecology*, 3, 157–161.

GRAHAM, H. (1976) 'Smoking in pregnancy: the attitudes of expectant mothers', *Social Science and Medicine*, 10, 399–405.

GRAHAM, H. (1985) *Caring for the Family*, Faculty of Social Sciences, Milton Keynes, Open University.

GRAHAM, H. (1987) 'Women's smoking and family health', *Social Science and Medicine*, 25(1), 47–56.

GRAHAM, H. (1988) 'Women and smoking in the United Kingdom: the implications for health promotion', *Health Promotion*, 3(4), 371–82.

GRAHAM, H. (1993a) *When Life's a Drag: Women, Smoking and Disadvantage*, London, HMSO.

GRAHAM, H. (1993b) *Hardship and Health in Women's Lives*, London, Harvester Wheatsheaf.

GRAHAM, H. and HUNT, S. (1994) 'Women's smoking and measures of women's socio-economic status in the United Kingdom', *Health Promotion*, 9(2), 81–8.

HOUSE OF COMMONS (1991) *Low Income Statistics: Households Below Average Income Tables*, London, HMSO.

JACKSON, R. and BENGLEHOLE, R. (1985) 'Secular trends in under-reporting of cigarette consumption', *American Journal of Epidemiology*, 122, 341–44.

JACOBSON, B. (1986) *Beating the Ladykillers*, London, Pluto Press.

JARVIS, M. (1984) 'Gender and smoking: do women really find it harder to give up?', *British Journal of Addiction*, 79, 57–61.

JARVIS, M. and JOHNSON, P. (1988) 'Cigar and pipe smoking in Britain: implications for smoking prevalence and cessation', *British Journal of Addiction*, 83, 103–110.

KIERNAN, K. (1992) 'Men and women at work and at home' in JOWELL, R., BROOK, L., PRIOR, G. and TAYLOR, B. (Eds) *British Social Attitudes: the 9th Report*, Aldershot, Dartmouth.

LADER, D. and MATHESON, J. (1991) *Smoking Among Secondary School Children in 1990*, London, HMSO.

MADLEY, R. J., GILLIES, P. A., POWER, F. L. and SYMONDS, E. M. (1989) 'Nottingham Mothers Stop Smoking Project — baseline survey of smoking in pregnancy', *Community Medicine*, **11**(2), 124–30.

MARSH, A. and MATHESON, J. (1983) *Smoking Attitudes and Behaviour*, London, HMSO.

MCKENNELL, A. C. and THOMAS, R. K. (1967) *Adults' and Adolescents' Smoking Habits and Attitudes*, London, HMSO.

NICOTINELL (1993) *Smoking Mothers with Young Children: The Hidden Dilemma*, London, Nicotinell.

OAKLEY, A. (1979) *Becoming a Mother*, Martin Robertson, Oxford.

OAKLEY, A. (1989) 'Smoking in pregnancy: smokescreen or risk factor? Towards a materialist analysis', *Sociology of Health and Illness*, **11**(4), 311–335.

OAKLEY, A., BRANNEN, J. and DODD, K. (1992) 'Young people, gender and smoking in the United Kingdom', *Health Promotion International*, **7**(2), 75–88.

OFFICE OF POPULATION CENSUSES AND SURVEYS (OPCS) (1992) *General Household Survey 1990*, London, HMSO.

OLDFIELD, N. and YU, A. C. S. (1993) *The Cost of A Child*, London, CPAG.

PAHL, R. E. (1984) *Divisions of Labour*, Oxford, Blackwell.

PETO, R., LOPEZ, A. D., BOREHAM, J., THUN, M. and HEATH, C. (1992) 'Mortality from tobacco in developed countries: indirect estimation from national vital statistics', *The Lancet*, **339**, 268–78.

PIERCE, J. P. (1989) 'International comparisons in trends in cigarette smoking prevalence', *AJPH*, **79**(2), 152–7.

ROYAL COLLEGE OF PHYSICIANS (1992) *Smoking and the Young*, a report of a working party of the Royal College of Physicians, London, Royal College of Physicians.

SECRETARY OF STATE FOR HEALTH (1992) *Health of the Nation: A Strategy for Health in England*, London, HMSO.

SIMMS, M. and SMITH, C. (1986) *Teenage Mothers and Their Partners*, London, HMSO.

TODD, G. F. (1978) 'Cigarette consumption per adult of each sex in various countries', *Journal of Epidemiology and Community Health*, **32**, 285–33.

TOWNSEND, P. DAVIDSON, N. and WHITEHEAD, M. (1988) *Inequalities in Health*, London, Penguin.

WALD, N., KIRYLUK, S., DARBY, S., DOLL, R., PIKE, M. and PETO, R. (1988) *UK Smoking Statistics*, Oxford, Oxford University Press.

WELLS, J. (1987) *Women and Smoking: an Evaluation of the Role of Stress in Smoking Cessation and Relapse*, Southampton, Department of Psychology, University of Southampton.

WHITE, A., FREETH, S. and O'BRIEN, M. (1992) *Infant Feeding 1990*, London, HMSO.

WILKINSON, R. (1989) 'Class mortality differentials, income distribution and trends in poverty, 1921–81', *Journal of Social Policy*, **18**(3), 307–36.

Chapter 8

Towards a Feminist Approach to Breast Cancer

Sue Wilkinson and Celia Kitzinger

Breast Cancer: A Feminist Issue

It is a central tenet of feminism that women's invisible private wounds often reflect social and political injustices. It is a commitment central to feminism to share burdens. And it is an axiom of feminism that the personal is political. (Datan, 1989, p. 175)

Nancy Datan, the feminist psychologist now dead from breast cancer, who wrote these words, was calling for the development of feminist theory and practice around the issue of breast cancer. In this chapter we look in more detail at the harm that is done to women with breast cancer both by orthodox medicine and by alternative philosophies of 'self-help'. We then sketch out some of the main features which we see as essential to developing a feminist approach to breast cancer and its 'treatment'.

Breast cancer is a major health issue for women: there are 22,000 cases per year in England and Wales (OPCS *Cancer Statistics* for 1985, published 1990). One in twelve of us develops breast cancer at some point in our lives and it is the leading cause of death for women in the 45–64 age group. For lesbians, the risk of breast cancer is even higher because fewer of us have borne children: the incidence of breast cancer is about doubled for women who postpone childbearing until after the age of thirty, or who do not have children (MacMahon, 1970, quoted in Travis, 1988).

Breast cancer is not just physically traumatic, but also causes tremendous emotional distress. Jo Spence, the feminist photographer, diagnosed as having breast cancer (and who has since died) writes about how 'I have had to face the fact that I am totally vulnerable, able to die, to feel terror, to be terrorized' (Spence, 1986). Many women seriously consider killing themselves during the period of physical recovery from mastectomy (25 per cent in one study: Wellisch *et al.*, 1978). Few women feel they are getting adequate support from their family and friends: in one study more than half said the support was inadequate and nearly three-quarters said that other people seemed to avoid and fear them (Peters-Golden, 1982). And, indeed, other people do: 61 per cent of healthy people say they might avoid contact with a friend who had cancer (Peters-Golden, 1982).

Male Constructions and Medical Practice

The experience of breast cancer is clearly influenced by the cultural emphasis on breasts as objects of male sexual interest and male sexual pleasure:

> Given that women are expected to be the object of the male gaze, are expected to beautify themselves in order to become loveable, are still fighting for basic rights over their own bodies, it seemed to me that the breast could be seen as a metaphor for our struggles . . . (Spence, 1986, p. 155).

The 'page 3' mentality is reproduced in the medical and psychological literature, as well as in the material from major cancer charities. In one advertisement, two images are juxtaposed: a shadowed breast and a perfect, luscious pear. Superimposed on the breast, around the nipple, are three dotted circles, containing the instruction 'press'. Breast self-examination is trivialised in the manner of a smutty seaside postcard. The illustrations for a breast self-examination leaflet produced by the Women's National Cancer Control Campaign (reproduced in Baum, 1988) are indistinguishable from soft porn. The conventionally attractive, slim, white model poses coyly, self-consciously stroking her large 'perfect' breasts.

The routine use in the medical literature of words like 'disfigurement', 'mutilation' and 'lop-sided' to describe the post-mastectomy patient both reinforces women's own sense of their bodily imperfections and reflects men's horror at wounded female bodies. Throughout the medical and psychological literature, the implicit assumption is that women's breasts are there for men's sexual pleasure. When women express concern about the loss of their breasts, this is frequently trivialised: 'no one will know' or 'we can make you a new one'. One woman who was told she would have to have a mastectomy recounts how her surgeon broke the news: 'It's not the end of the world', he beamed, 'I can make you another one. If you were my wife, I'd want you to have it' (Prior, 1987, p. 920).

There seems to be more concern about the effect of the mastectomy on the women's husbands than on the women themselves. One advertisement, portraying a worried-looking man, asks: 'How would a mastectomy affect your other half?'. The text continues: 'A woman's breast cancer can seriously affect someone else. Her partner... Macmillan Breast Care nurses talk at length about their loved one's cancer...'.

Despite the heterosexism of this advert, many men do find breast cancer distressing — about half the women in one study said that their husbands found looking at their scar distressing (Meyerowitz, 1981, cited in Meyerowitz *et al.*, 1988) — and psychologists have developed 'treatment' for such men, including 'systematic desensitisation', which entails deep relaxation as steadily more distressing scenarios are presented in sequence (Tarrier and Maguire, 1984).

The medical profession is especially concerned to ensure that men have sexual intercourse with their post-mastectomy wives. This is, in fact, part of what is meant by 'normalisation of life to pre-mastectomy status'. Women who have had mastectomies are diagnosed as suffering from 'sexual dysfunction' if they have 'stopped intercourse or ceased to enjoy it' (Maguire, 1978). The restrictedness of this definition and its offensiveness to all women — especially lesbians — is self-evident. Moreover, sometimes women themselves are not even consulted about their sexuality. In one study, the husbands of mastectomy patients were asked about their overall sexual satisfaction and about the frequency with which their wives submitted to sexual intercourse (Wellisch *et al.*, 1978).

Mastectomy and After

The emphasis on sexuality and body image — meaning being attractive to men and engaging in sexual intercourse with them — is a major preoccupation of the psychiatric and psychological literature on mastectomy. There is very little discussion of other issues in relation to breast loss — breast feeding, or explaining (or concealing) the loss of a breast to a child, for example.

Treatment of women post-mastectomy focuses on encouraging

women to 'look feminine' as quickly as possible (Meyerowitz *et al.*, 1988). Nurses are told to help women to do their hair nicely and apply make-up while still in their hospital beds (Anstice, 1970; Byrd, 1975).

Prostheses are fitted as soon as possible. A prosthesis is a false breast made of lambswool to be stuffed inside a bra, or a breast-shaped pocket to serve as a substitute breast. These (according to the North American 'Reach to Recovery' booklet) can be weighted with birdseed, rice, small plastic beads, fishing sinkers or gunshot. Eventually, women are fitted with prostheses made of plastic, silicon or rubber. In the UK, NHS prostheses are marketed with names like 'Carefree', 'Tru Life' and 'Confidante' (Baum, 1988). In the USA, there is one called 'Nearly Me', marketed by Ruth Handler, described as 'the woman who . . . dared to put bosoms on Barbie Doll' (cf. Daly, 1979).

Discomfort in wearing a prosthesis is a commonly reported physical complaint following mastectomy. Yet the message a woman gets in the first morning after surgery is to 'get fitted'. The message for a woman who has just had a mastectomy is that her body is now defective, and that her first priority is to seek an artificial cosmetic remedy, a lifetime of disguise. There is little room for accepting the loss of a breast, the wound, and the scar that healing will bring.

Increasingly, here and in the USA, so-called 'breast reconstruction' is heavily marketed. This involves taking new skin and tissue from another part of a woman's body and, keeping the blood vessels intact, these are swung around to form a mound on the site of the original breast. Alternatively, the breast tissue can be substituted by a plastic sac which is laced under the skin and then filled with fluid until the 'correct' size is reached (Fallowfield, 1991).

Twenty thousand women in the USA undergo breast reconstruction each year. No wonder — when post-mastectomy patients in the USA are routinely given, on the day after the mastectomy, a leaflet written by the American Society of Plastic and Reconstructive Surgeons, Inc. It says:

> If you are like most women, your breasts have great psychological significance to you and you will feel more feminine and more secure socially and sexually with a reconstructed breast following mastectomy for cancer (Datan, 1989, p. 181).

Breast reconstruction does not, of course, restore sensation to a breast, the implant can result in heavy bleeding and infection, and further surgery may be needed if it shifts position. After a breast reconstruction, recurrences of cancer on the chest wall are much harder to detect. Michael Baum, Professor of Surgery at the Royal Marsden Hospital has said recently that a main goal of breast reconstruction is 'to establish symmetry between the new breast mound and the remaining breast' (Baum, 1988). He also says 'this may entail reduction mammoplasty for the other side': in other words, they chop bits off the healthy breast to make it 'match' the reconstructed one — most likely for women with large breasts, bigger than a size B bra cup. Baum also aims 'to create a pleasing nipple/areola complex' — he does NOT mention that this may entail using skin from the remaining nipple or from the labia (Faulder, 1989). The language used in the medical literature in discussing breast reconstruction is all about exciting new medical advances to improve on women's bodies. They write, for example, of 'ingenious new techniques' to enable 'the exhibition of a modest degree of cleavage' (Baum, 1988).

How far can these preoccupations be taken? One woman tells of the pressure put on her, following mastectomy and breast reconstruction, to have a second mastectomy (of her healthy breast) — and of her regrets:

> My own second mastectomy, performed at the time of breast reconstruction, was prophylactic. My surgeon said he could not offer 'a good match' after reconstruction unless both breasts were reconstructed and I allowed myself to be swayed to his belief. Now, I regret sacrificing my healthy left breast . . . If I had to do it again, I would not trade a healthy, functioning breast just to try to achieve what a surgeon calls 'a better match'. It is a lasting regret. I could have breastfed our son if I had resisted that surgeon's coercion . . . (Johnson, 1987, p. 101).

If these examples seem incredibly offensive, it is worth pointing out that even the most cursory glance at the breast cancer literature yields many more examples of this kind. Of course, we are not suggesting that such instances should debar women from seeking needed medical help. But such attitudes and practices reflect assumptions and values widely held within the culture, so it is perhaps not surprising that we have found the psychological and medical literature redolent with sexism and heterosexism. Nor are we saying that (the few) feminists — particularly sociologists — working in cancer medicine have failed to offer a critique of its man-made orthodoxy (e.g., Morris, 1983), or its disregard and distortion of women's experience (e.g., Rosser, 1991). However, it is clear that these lone voices remain largely unheard in the medical wilderness.

Heal Thyself: 'Alternative' Health Care

What the 'Self-help' Books Say

The medical profession, at best, denies women power; at the worst, it reduces us to the state of passive victims. Feeling this loss of control, this passivity and powerlessness in men's hands, and desperate to 'do something' about their illness, it is little wonder that many women turn to the complementary, fringe or holistic health care movements, which appear to offer women a measure of control and power over their lives. Many women are now involved in these. When Sue O'Sullivan co-ordinated a day workshop on 'Women, Health and Sexuality' at an adult education institute she was not prepared for:

> ...the number of women who were so wound up in holistic medicine that reactions to oppression and exploitation, as well as health, were individualised into a matter of a 'state of mind'. Not only could you prevent cancer through being 'in tune' with your mind and body, you could transcend sexism by the same method (O'Sullivan, 1984, p. 51).

Because we are psychologists, we have looked particularly at the psychological claims made by many of the popular 'self-help' books and tapes available for women with cancer. The basic argument of these books and tapes is that we give ourselves cancer because of unhealthy attitudes, personality or behaviour — and that we can get rid of it by developing positive thinking and/or a healthier lifestyle.

Such ideas are, in fact, neither 'new' nor 'alternative': as long ago as 200 AD the Roman physician Galen had observed that 'melancholic' women were more likely to get breast cancer than 'sanguine' women, and the association between cancer and certain 'mental dispositions' can be traced on through histories of medicine (Brohn, 1987). It is certainly part of current medical orthodoxy, as indicated in a 1991 article in the British Medical Journal:

> Certain personality traits, such as tendency to suppress emotion, especially anger, and to respond to stress by using a repressive coping style, have been found to be commoner in patients with cancer (Lovestone and Fahy, 1991, p. 1219).

Ellen Goudsmit and Robin Gadd (1991) present a compelling argument for the 'psychologising' of women's physical illness as typical.

There is a plethora of popular and semi-popular books and tapes available for the cancer sufferer. We will look at how the arguments are developed in three widely-read 'self-help manuals' — Penny Brohn's *The Bristol Programme*; Rachael Clyne's *Cancer — Your Life, Your Choice*; and Colin Ryder Richardson's *Mind over Cancer* — and in a tape by Louise Hay called *Cancer — Discovering Your Healing Power*. This tape is a bestseller at feminist bookshops (we got it at Silver Moon in London). These books and tapes exude an aura of warmth and hope: they talk of nature, spirituality, and love; their covers depict rainbows (Richardson), leaves (Brohn), hearts (Hay) and a circle of people with linked arms (Clyne). All take an holistic view of health and illness:

> Cancer can be broadly viewed as the result of decreasing co-operation with the natural flow of life (Clyne, 1989, p. 60).

> Cancer or similar diseases are illnesses of the weakened spirit which is off balance and has lost the rhythm of life, of love (Richardson, 1988, p. 105).

These books and tapes say we are responsible for giving ourselves cancer; that we can cure ourselves of it; that we can choose whether to get well or not; that it is our own fault if we die. Individual, personal responsibility at every step is the overwhelming message of the 'self-help' literature.

Louise Hay's tape says we cause cancer by our thoughts and beliefs:

> It is my belief that we are each 100 per cent responsible for every experience in our lives — the best and the worst. We all create our experiences by the thoughts we think and the words we speak. The universe totally supports us in every thought we choose to think and believe. Our subconscious mind accepts whatever we choose to believe ... And we have unlimited choice about what we can think ... Resentment, criticism and guilt are the most damaging mental thought patterns we can have. This kind of thinking creates and maintains dis-ease in the body. Acid, biting thoughts often create acid blood and your blood is your life force. These thoughts literally eat away at the body. Criticism as a permanent habit can often lead to arthritis. Guilt always looks for punishment and creates pain. And resentment, long held, eats away at the body and becomes the dis-ease we call cancer (Hay, 1984).

For Colin Richardson, 'negative attitudes' lead to 'negative behaviour patterns', which in turn damage the body:

> Perhaps you are young and have breast cancer — so why have you got this illness? Have you been on the pill? Have you had affairs of the heart too often? If you have been a mother, have you naturally breast fed your children? Has your past life been totally blameless? Haven't you somehow abused yourself sexually? Most cancers are preventable and are found mainly in persons guilty of self-abuse. Just know that cancers are far less common in disciplined societies — it is for example rare for nuns to have cancer of the neck of the womb . . . (Richardson, 1988, pp. 100–101).

Richardson's misogyny continues as he suggests husbands may have cancer because their wives drink, shoplift, or are 'unfaithful'; and children may have cancer because their mothers smoked while pregnant.

Responsible for causing our cancer, we must take personal responsibility for getting rid of it. All that is needed is to harness the power of positive thought:

> The first step usually involves coming to terms with our reality; being willing to accept our feelings and circumstances exactly as they are, without condition. Strangely enough this in itself can produce a powerful sense of freedom — a change in the way that we experience something that takes the burden or significance of it away. Accepting a point of view of responsibility then begins to create this opportunity of choice, the opportunity that we can choose to experience our situation another way (Clyne, 1989, pp. 84–5).

The next step is to 'let go' of negative patterns of thought:

> When we want to begin to change a condition, one of the first things to do is to say so. Literally say 'I am willing to release that pattern within me that is creating this experience or condition'. You can say this to yourself over and over every time you think of your illness . . . The minute you say it you are stepping out of the victim role. You are no longer helpless. You are acknowledging your own power (Hay, 1984).

We must forgive our abusers, accept life exactly as it is and — particularly — offer ourselves total and unconditional love:

> If we are open to the giving and receiving of love we are becoming part of the most powerful force in the universe . . .

... As we learn more and more about love we will find that it is actually possible to handle everything that comes our way with love. Gradually we shall have less need to respond with anger, fear, grief or sympathy because, by understanding these emotions better we shall gain control over them. Once we have achieved this we can choose to detach from these responses and use only love (Brohn, 1987, p. 130).

No negative condition can remain in our lives when we truly love and accept ourselves. Love is the healing force. Love dissolves anger. Love gets rid of guilt. Love fades away fear. Love for ourselves is the power that heals us (Hay, 1984).

There is no need to change any situation, only our reaction to it — and it is also made quite clear that if we cannot do this, it is our own fault that we remain ill:

When we first started the Centre one of our earliest patients was a girl with lung secondaries following a breast cancer. She was enthusiastic about what Bristol had to offer, was a vigorous and faithful devotee of the diet, had her doctor running around prescribing all the vitamins and minerals, and was generally a model patient. Unfortunately, she did not seem to be much better for all this, and we were concerned about her lack of progress... it became clear that this girl had such a low self-image that she couldn't do such a thing as picture herself well and happy. I believe that if people have such a low self-image they cannot even IMAGINE themselves better, then no amount of treatment in the world can help them (Brohn, 1987, p. 144).

The logic of this extends even to making us responsible for our own death: 'Your mind is very powerful and if you feel you are going to die, you will. It is as simple as that' (Richardson, 1988, p. 95). We may even positively 'choose' to die:

... a very small number of people ... had cancer for a slightly different reason ... They all died and I believe they chose to have cancer as a means of growing spiritually, the benefits of which went beyond Death ... One ... had to go through the process of dying for what he described as his 'group spirit' to evolve. Another had expressed his certainty of reincarnation and implied that his illness was a major growing point in his own continuum (Clyne, 1989, pp. 88–9).

If we do not choose death, some of these programmes promise a cure for cancer: Louise Hay's is intended to 'build perfect, vibrant health', which she sees as 'our birthright'. Others make a clear distinction between physical and mental 'healing':

> Some patients... are glaringly aware of the fact that the cancer has not gone away. It is still palpable and painful, and they are actually conscious of it. Nevertheless... finish up with a mental picture of being clear and free from disease. We believe that this is important on levels of other than the physical. We shall all be completely healed in a spiritual sense, whether or not we get rid of the disease (Brohn, 1987, pp. 141–2).

However, all offer some version of wholeness, happiness, growth, joy, enlightenment, fulfilment or empowerment, which is attained by the exercise of freedom, control and choice:

> ...learn to redraw the rules of life in your favour. This is natural freedom to which we are all entitled... I have made these changes and because of them I AM GLAD I HAD CANCER!...

> I have a freedom that previously I did not possess. This freedom is entirely in the brain. It means I can enjoy life better by accepting the good things we all have and rejecting the bad things we don't require... worries are now rejected and instead a feeling of warm love is within me (Richardson, 1988, p. 134).

This message is a dangerous one for the distressed and desperate cancer sufferer. It is full of false promises; it indulges in victim-blaming of the highest order; and it offers a spurious illusion of power over illness, indeed over all aspects of life. It does not admit to any causes of cancer over which we may have no control, and it takes no account of the material realities of most women's lives. Christabelle Sethna (1992) criticises a similar message on New Age 'subliminal persuasion/self-hypnosis' tapes marketed to 'release' women from the effects of pre-menstrual syndrome, abortion, and sexual abuse.

Why They Say It

While it is clear what the 'alternative' therapies offer the cancer patient, why does their broad philosophy appear to be so widely accepted in western society? Susan Sontag provides an explanation both in terms of the history of medicine and the contemporary popularity of psychology:

> ... theories that diseases are caused by mental states and can be cured by will power are always an index of how much is not understood about the physical terrain of a disease. Moreover, there is a peculiarly modern predeliction for psychological explanations of disease, as of everything else. Psychologising seems to provide control over the experiences and events (like grave illnesses) over which people have in fact little or no control (Sontag, 1979, p. 56).

She goes on to show how the nineteenth century psychologising of tuberculosis evaporated with the advent of streptomycin; psychological analysis now surrounds the twentieth century diseases of cancer and HIV/AIDS.

It is not coincidental that these diseases are often viewed within a moral context. As Rosalind Coward argues, western society (and, we would add, western psychology) has long sustained a view of an individual 'self' or 'inner core' of personality which determines behaviour and experience. She continues:

> In particular, there has always been an attempt to link this view of the personality to morality, to the existence of good and bad people. Everything which happens to an individual is ultimately to be explained by their own actions and therefore their personal responsibility. It is not hard to see the ways in which this has been translated into the body and health, where the whole person is the person who will not become ill, and the unharmonious individual is the one who will be susceptible to disease ... It is as if disease has become a kind of morality, demonstrating the level of the individual's control over their life (Coward, 1989, p. 92).

In the twentieth century, capitalist economy, redolent with Thatcherite values, health as one's personal responsibility (and moral duty) is a very convenient rhetoric. As Carol Smith (1980) points out, although many cancers are thought to be caused by the conditions under which we work, government publications typically play down occupational factors and emphasise the need for people to 'look after their own health'. They argue that we 'voluntarily' expose ourselves to cancer risk, for example by smoking or by eating an 'unhealthy' diet. Alternative medicine's attempts to get people to take individual responsibility only reinforce such a victim-blaming approach.

Towards a Feminist Theory of Breast Cancer

Orthodox medical and 'alternative' approaches to breast cancer are both harmful to women. We need to move beyond them to develop a feminist theory of breast cancer. Of course, such a theory is not a freestanding alternative to traditional or complementary medicine. The physical realities of breast cancer will usually necessitate engagement with a range of medical practices — and we are not simply suggesting the substitution of sisterhood for surgery. However, a feminist theory of breast cancer cannot mean accepting male definitions of our 'femininity' and sexuality, or victim-blaming fantasies of omnipotence over the cause of our disease. We must lay claim to our experience of breast cancer through, for example, consciousness-raising, and we must develop a thoroughgoing politics of illness which incorporates industrial society's contribution to ill-health, and analyses the social and economic forces that frame the availability and 'choice' of 'treatments' for cancer. Further, we cannot stop at theory: we need to develop feminist practice around breast cancer, through, for example, political lobbying and the provision of illness support groups. Here we illustrate how such theory and practice may be developed, largely through the words of women who have spoken out about the meaning of breast cancer for their own lives and feminist politics.

To begin with, we must acknowledge that 'silence and invisibility go hand in hand with powerlessness' (Smith, 1980, p. vii), and that breast cancer must be publicly 'owned' as an issue for ALL of us within the feminist community. As Nancy Datan writes:

> The woman who has been raped or might be, the mother seeking child care, or the woman seeking an abortion, all face issues that once were defined as personal and private and now are seen as public and political. Breast cancer too can be seen as more than a singular affliction, as feminists consider rape to be not an isolated personal trauma but an expression of a larger social context in which male sexuality, the patriarchal family, and aggression against women are blended. Similarly, breast cancer is not a solitary ordeal but an illness of the community, to which the community responds with an expression of communal values, which may certainly include repudiation, denial and isolation (Datan, 1989, pp. 183–4).

Repudiation, denial and isolation cannot be overcome until we can speak freely of our experience, whether we are the friends and lovers of those with breast cancer, or have had breast cancer ourselves. Feminist writers such as Audre Lorde (1980, 1982), Adrienne Rich (1978) and Nancy Datan (1989), in speaking out about the experience of breast cancer, enable others to speak out also, and to expose the hetero-patriarchal values inherent in both orthodox medical and 'alternative' treatments for breast cancer. Visual images, too, have prompted feminist reappraisals of the meanings of our breasts and the violence perpetuated by men in the 'treatment' of breast cancer (e.g., Spence, 1986; Sebestyen, 1992).

As feminists we need to expose silicon implants as 'a clear example of how both sexism and the profit motive effect women's lives' (Smith, 1980); take issue with the pernicious practice of victim-blaming; and seek to identify — and, as far as we can, *prevent* — causes of cancer largely unacknowledged by those in power. Of course, neither we nor the medical profession know the full story about what causes cancer, but our levels of explanation — and priorities for action — are likely to be very different. Jackie Winnow, a longtime lesbian-feminist activist and founder of the Women's Cancer Resource Center in Berkeley, California (who died of breast cancer in 1991) writes:

> Real prevention would mean changing fundamental social structures. It would mean going after the tobacco industry, stopping the pollution of our environment, providing quality food. But when the medical profession talks about prevention, they mean at best small, individual acts — like stopping smoking and reducing dietary fat intake. When they talk about prevention, they talk about early detection methods like mammograms or breast self-examination. But once a tumour is found in your breast, you already have cancer ... (Winnow, 1992, p. 73).

Audre Lorde, in her powerful account of her own experience of breast cancer, sees the effects of victim-blaming — and environmental pollution — on her own life:

> Last week I read a letter from a doctor in a medical magazine which said that no truly happy person ever gets cancer. Despite my knowing better, and despite my having dealt with this blame-the-victim thinking for years, for a moment this letter hit my guilt button. Had I really been guilty of the crime of not being happy in this best of all possible infernos? ...
> Was I wrong to be working so hard against the oppressions

afflicting women and Black people? Was I in error to be speaking out against our silent passivity and the cynicism of a mechanised and inhuman civilization that is destroying our earth and those who live upon it? Was I really fighting the spread of radiation, racism, woman-slaughter, chemical invasion of our food, pollution of our environment, the abuse and psychic destruction of our young, merely to avoid dealing with my first and greatest responsibility — to be happy? . . .

The happiest person in this country cannot help breathing in smokers' cigarette fumes, auto exhaust, and airborne chemical dust, nor avoid drinking the water, and eating the food. The idea that happiness can insulate us against the results of our environmental madness is a rumour circulated by our enemies to destroy us . . . We are equally destroyed by false happiness and false breasts, and the passive acceptance of false values which corrupt our lives and distort our experience (Lorde, 1980, pp. 66–7).

Reflecting the false notion of 'survivor', some women claim their own victimhood. A lesbian with pervasive cancers in different sites of her body identifies herself as:

. . . a victim of the government's irresponsible bombing experiments in the Nevada desert. Here I was victim of fall-out when I was just a teenager and stood outside watching the beautiful yellow sky. My sisters (I have five) began, now, to get cancer. My older sister and the one just younger than me. Did we three stand under the same yellow sky, or did we drink the same contaminated milk or chew on a blade of grass thick with poisons: rolling on the lawn on hot summer nights after the big mushroom's death particles bathed our homes and gardens with 'safe-level fall-out'? (Johnson, 1981, p. 8).

Such experience must be shared within our feminist communities. It must be analysed within a feminist political framework — and such analyses must be turned into political action.

In the USA, feminist activists have pointed to the discrepancy between resources available for AIDS and for cancer, given the relative scale of these problems for women: e.g., in 1988, there were 100 women with AIDS in the San Francisco Bay Area, and approximately 40,000 with cancer (Winnow, 1992). The national Women's Health Network (an organization which promotes and monitors women's health-care delivery in the USA) has testified at Congressional hearings that the government must reconsider its current priority of funding research for treatment while ignoring research for prevention (Rosen, 1991). Women with breast cancer have started organisations to lobby for better preventative care, increased research funding and improved insurance coverage; and to provide information and support services for all women whose lives are touched by breast cancer. Examples of such organisations are the Women's Cancer Resource Center, Berkeley, California; the Women's Community Cancer Project, Cambridge, Massachusetts (both of which provide a mix of political action, education, information and support services); and the Mautner Project for Lesbians With Cancer, Washington DC (which proves direct services to lesbians with cancer, their families, and caregivers).

Fostering a sense of feminist community is central to the philosophy of all of these projects. This is perhaps seen most clearly in their establishment of support groups which do not exist in order to swell the plastic surgeon's profits (as in Reach to Recovery), but which provide women with personal and practical resources to face the trauma of breast cancer AND the strength to challenge male power. Describing one such lesbian support group, Joan Nestle writes:

> The group does not make illness go away, it does not bring back breasts or vision or the ability to walk without pain, but it tells me that in other lesbian lives the struggle goes on, and when I see their power and courage I am close to the heart of everything that has given my life meaning — the lesbian spirit of defiance and creation (Nestle, 1981, p. 8).

Nancy Johnson was a member of this group and was supported by it in her class action suit against the US government for condemning the people of Utah to years of cancer.

One of the important attractions of the alternative health movement is that it offers us the illusion of 'stepping out of the victim role' (Hay, 1984). By contrast, a feminist analysis of health and illness begins by acknowledging that we ARE victims — victims of a patriarchal world and a heterosexist health system, which, as feminists, we struggle against. It continues with campaigns and community action: to change current medical, social and political approaches to cancer, and to provide information and support for all who need it. That is what 'stepping out of the victim role' really means. That is what we mean by a feminist approach to breast cancer.

Notes

1   An earlier version of this chapter appeared in *Women's Studies International Forum* (1993), **16**(3), 229–238.
2   We would like to thank Susan Liroff of the Women's Cancer Resource Center, Berkeley, for her help.

References

ANSTICE, E. (1970) Coping after a mastectomy, *Nursing Times*, **66**, 882–3.

BAUM, M. (1988) *Breast Cancer: The Facts*, 2nd Edition, Oxford, Oxford University Press.

BROHN, P. (1987) *The Bristol Programme: An Introduction to the Holistic Therapies Practised by the Bristol Cancer Help Centre*, London, Century.

BYRD, B. F. (1975) 'Sex after mastectomy', *Medical Aspects of Human Sexuality*, **9**(4), 53–4.

CLYNE, R. (1989) *Cancer — Your Life, Your Choice*, Wellingborough, Thorsons.

COWARD, R. (1989) *The Whole Truth: The Myth of Alternative Health*, London, Faber and Faber.

DALY, M. (1979) *Gyn/Ecology: The Metaethics of Radical Feminism*, London, The Women's Press.

DATAN, N. (1989) 'Illness and imagery: Feminist cognition, socialization and gender identity', in CRAWFORD, M. and GENTRY, M. (Eds) *Gender and Thought: Psychological Perspectives*, New York, Springer-Verlag.

FALLOWFIELD, L. with CLARK, A. (1991) *Breast Cancer*, London, Tavistock/Routledge.

FAULDER, C. (1989) *The Women's Cancer Book*, London, Virago.

GOUDSMIT, E. M. and GADD, R. (1991) 'All in the mind? The psychologisation of illness', *The Psychologist, The Bulletin of the British Psychological Society*, **14**(10), 449–453.

HAY, L. (1984) *Cancer — Discovering Your Healing Power*, (Tape) Santa Monica, CA, Hay House Inc.

JOHNSON, J. E. (1987) *Intimacy: Living as a Woman After Cancer*, Toronto, NC Press Ltd.

JOHNSON, N. (1981) 'The dragon-slayer', *Off Our Backs*, **6**(5), 8.

LORDE, A. (1980) *The Cancer Journals*, London, Sheba Feminist Publishers.

LORDE, A. (1982) *Zami: A New Spelling of My Name*, London, Sheba Feminist Publishers.

LOVESTONE, S. and FAHY, T. (1991) 'Psychological factors in breast cancer', *British Medical Journal*, **302**, 25 May, 1219–20.

MAGUIRE, P. (1978) 'Psychiatric problems after mastectomy', in BRAND, P. C. and VAN KEEP, P. A. (Eds) *Breast Cancer: Psycho-social Aspects of Early Detection and Treatment*, Baltimore, MD, University Park Press.

MEYEROWITZ, B. E., CHAIKEN, S. and CLARK, L. K. (1988) 'Sex roles and culture: Social and personal reactions to breast cancer', in FINE, M. and ASCH, A. (Eds) *Women With Disabilities: Essays in Psychology, Culture and Politics*, Philadelphia, Temple University Press.

MORRIS, T. (1983) 'Psycho-social aspects of breast cancer: a review', *European Journal of Cancer and Clinical Oncology*, **19**(12), 1725–1735.

NESTLE, J. (1981) 'New York lesbian illness support group: what being a lesbian means in the deepest sense', *Off Our Backs*, **6**(5), 7–8.

OPCS (1990) *Cancer Statistics: Registrations 1985*, London, HMSO.

O'SULLIVAN, S. (1984) 'Patients and power', *Trouble and Strife*, **3**, Summer, 50–53.

PETERS-GOLDEN, H. (1982) 'Breast cancer: varied perceptions of social support in the illness experience', *Social Science and Medicine*, **16**, 482–491.

PRIOR, A. (1987) 'Personal View' *British Medical Journal*, **295**, 10 October, 920.

RICH, A. (1978) *The Dream of a Common Language: Poems 1974–1977*, New York, W. W. Norton and Co.

RICHARDSON, C. R. (1988) *Mind Over Cancer*, London, W. Foulsham and Co. Ltd.

ROSEN, R. (1991) 'Breast cancer: An ignored epidemic', *University of California at Davis Magazine*, Spring, 17.

ROSSER, J. E. (1991) 'The interpretation of women's experience: A critical appraisal of the literature on breast cancer', *Social Science and Medicine*, **15E**, 257–265.

SEBESTYEN, A. (1992) 'The cancer drawings of Catherine Arthur', *Feminist Review*, **No 41**, Summer, 27–36.

SETHNA, C. (1992) 'Accepting "total and complete responsibility": New Age neo-feminist violence against women', *Feminism and Psychology: An International Journal*, **2**(1), 113–119.

SMITH, C. (1980) Foreword to the first British edition of Audre Lorde's *The Cancer Journals*, London, Sheba Feminist Publishers.

SONTAG, S. (1979) *Illness as Metaphor*, London, Allen Lane.

SPENCE, J. (1986) *Putting Myself in the Picture: A Political, Personal and Photographic Autobiography*, London, Camden Press.

TARRIER, N. and MAGUIRE, P. (1984) 'Treatment of psychological distress following mastectomy: an initial report', *Behavioural Research and Therapy*, **22**, 81–84.

TRAVIS, C. B. (1988) *Women and Health: Biomedical Issues*, Hillsday, NJ, Lawrence Erlbaum.

WELLISCH, D. K., JAMISON, K. R. and PASNAU, R. O. (1978) 'Psychosocial aspects of mastectomy II: The man's perspective', *American Journal of Psychiatry*, **135**, 543–546.

WINNOW, J. (1992) 'Lesbians evolving health care: Cancer and AIDS', *Feminist Review*, No 41, Summer, 68–76.

Chapter 9

A 'Cure for All Ills'? Constructions of the Menopause and the Chequered Fortunes of Hormone Replacement Therapy

Kate Hunt

Why HRT is a Central Feminist Issue

The last two decades have witnessed dramatic fluctuations in the fortunes of hormone replacement therapy (HRT). Not only have overall prescriptions oscillated in a spectacular fashion, but constituent drugs and preferred modes of administration, and the underlying rationale and emphasis of appropriate indications for use, have changed. These changes have occurred partly in response to the expanding epidemiological evidence on aspects of the purported benefits and risks of the therapy, particularly in relation to longer term use.

However, 'hormones' occupy a powerful if uneasy position in our cultural repertoire of explanations of gender differences and 'gender-appropriate' behaviour. The provision of hormones to 'replace' those 'lost' after the menopause is the embodiment of the medicalization of the menopause. As such, it is intimately entwined with the social construction of gender and gender-appropriate behaviour. Since such conceptualizations are replete with notions of biological essentialism and ageist and heterosexist assumptions which fuel sexism, the image of the menopause as an 'oestrogen deficiency syndrome' and the images of femininity that are invoked to promote its use have implications for women of all ages. In this, and in relation to issues of medical control, there are strong parallels with other aspects of women's health, particularly those related to reproductive issues.

A major concern in feminism (both in relation to health and other issues) has been empowerment, and particularly the acquisition and dissemination of information which enables women to participate fully in decisions about their bodies. Notions of a 'woman's right to choose' have been central in debate and activism around childbirth (e.g. Kitzinger, 1992), access to abortion (e.g. Boyle, 1992) and rejections of compulsory heterosexuality (e.g. Wilkinson and Kitzinger, 1993). The valorization of women's own experiences in the face of competing medical definitions has been a dominant theme of second wave feminism. These notions pervade the popular, academic and (some parts of the) medical literature on HRT and the menopause in complex ways, and 'the' feminist position on HRT has been characterised as being very different on different sides of the Atlantic (McCrea and Markle, 1984).

The use of HRT thus raises and reflects important issues for a feminist agenda. This chapter discusses the current medical debate on HRT in the context of some of these broader issues. A summary of epidemiological evidence is presented first. Social constructions of the menopause are then addressed as one aspect of the prevalent tendency to dichotomize 'female' and 'male',[1] a tendency which commonly makes extensive recourse to biological essentialism for explanations.

A Brief History of HRT's Time: Patterns of Use and the Epidemiological Evidence

The debate within the medical literature on HRT (which has often been intense and polarized) has centred on two main themes: the consequences of use of HRT (and particularly long-term use) in relation to specific diseases; and appropriate indications for use. The main conditions or diseases to have received attention are osteoporosis, endometrial cancer (cancer of the lining of the womb), cardiovascular disease, and breast cancer. The main worries about adverse consequences of HRT have focused on endometrial and breast cancer and have generated concern and caution about the use of HRT, whilst evidence on reductions in the risk of osteoporosis and, more recently, cardiovascular disease have been the primary justifications for more widespread use of HRT as a preventive therapy. It is important when judging HRT from a public health perspective to be aware of the relative commoness of each of these diseases: in 1988, for example, all diseases of the circulatory system accounted for 90,958 deaths in women aged 45–84 years in England and Wales (with 49,216 deaths from ischaemic heart disease alone); equivalent figures for deaths attributed to breast and endometrial cancer were 10,995 and 805 respectively (see Hunt and Vessey, 1991a, p. 25).

The use of HRT to prevent osteoporosis led the way for a move from short-term prescribing to treat menopausal symptoms to prophylaxis. The prevention of osteoporosis (the development of brittle bones) has long been recognised as one indication for long-term use of HRT, although there is some controversy as to whether this should be restricted to women who are at 'high' risk of the disease. Several prospective studies (including some randomised control trials) have indicated that oestrogen is an effective means of preventing osteoporosis (see Hunt and Vessey, 1991a), although a number of factors are implicated in the aetiology of the condition. Reductions in risk of fractures of the hip and distal radius of around 50 per cent with five or more years use of oestrogens have typically been reported (Weiss *et al.*, 1980; Paganini-Hill *et al.*, 1981), particularly if use is started within five years of the menopause (Hutchinson *et al.*, 1979). It has been suggested that the greatest benefit is seen amongst women who have had their ovaries removed at a young age, and amongst recent or current users.

Endometrial Cancer

The first major worry about serious adverse effects of HRT which shook even the most hardened HRT enthusiasts was the publication in 1975 of the results of two case-control studies in a single issue of the *New England Journal of Medicine* (Smith *et al.*, 1975; Ziel and Finkle, 1975). These both reported that the risk of endometrial cancer was seven times higher amongst women who had taken unopposed HRT (that is, oestrogens alone) in comparison with women who had never taken HRT. These studies received widespread publicity, and the increase in oestrogen-associated cancers was described as 'one of the largest epidemics of serious iatrogenic disease that has ever occurred (in the USA)' (Jick *et al.*, 1980) with relative risks of 'a magnitude that has rarely been paralleled in the history of cancer reporting' (Weiss *et al.*, 1976). At least nineteen papers reporting results from case-control studies have been published since 1975, all but one of which have reported some elevation in risk (see Hunt and Vessey, 1987 and Hunt and Vessy, 1991a for details).

Some of the later papers were able to take account of methodological criticisms: it had been suggested that the earlier papers had exaggerated the level of risk either as a result of biases introduced by the selection of particular control groups, or because of possibilities of 'over-surveillance' or misdiagnosis in the oestrogen treated women.

On balance, and paying particular attention to studies published during the 1980s, it seems that the elevation in risk is between two-fold and four-fold when 'ever-users' of unopposed HRT are compared with 'never-users'. Several studies have reported risks for endometrial cancer which increase with increasing duration or dose (or both) of oestrogen use, but have suggested too that the increased risk is seen mainly for low-grade, early stage tumours with a good prognosis (although two recent studies have some evidence of increases in risk for more advanced disease (Shapiro *et al.*, 1985; Rubin *et al.*, 1990)).

The increase in risk of endometrial cancer associated with the use of unopposed oestrogens precipitated a change in prescribing practice. The dramatic effect on overall sales of HRT is described below, but in the early 1980s, it became increasingly common to prescribe a progestogen for women who had not had a hysterectomy. This drug regime (often referred to as combined or opposed therapy) was introduced following clinical studies which suggested that taking a progestogen for between ten and fourteen days in each four week cycle of oestrogen use eliminated or minimized the risk of endometrial cancer.[2] There are still few epidemiological data which relate to long-term use of opposed therapy, although a large cohort study in Sweden has indeed reported that there was no increase in endometrial cancer amongst women who had exclusively used opposed HRT (Persson *et al.*, 1989).

Breast Cancer

Whilst most disagreements about HRT and endometrial cancer have largely been resolved, in the 1980s and 1990s much of the focus of concern about iatrogenesis has shifted to breast cancer. The results of at least twenty case-control studies and eight cohort studies have been published since 1980 (see Hunt and Vessey, 1991b and Brinton and Schairer, 1993).

Although the data from these studies are less consistent than the numerous studies of endometrial cancer, on balance it seems that there is no increase in risk of breast cancer when 'ever-users' are compared with 'never-users'. However, a number of important uncertainties remain, notably, given the recent changes in prescribing patterns for HRT (i.e. more widespread use, recommendations for long-term prophylactic use, and more common use of opposed HRT; see below), the inadequate evidence on the effect of long durations of use and of opposed HRT. Most studies published since 1985 suggest that there may be an elevation in the risk of breast cancer with longer durations of use; one large American study, for example, reported a relative risk of 1.5 for twenty or more years of use of unopposed oestrogens (Brinton *et al.*, 1986), and a Swedish study has reported a doubling in risk with more than eight years' use (Bergkvist *et al.*, 1989). Four recent meta-analyses, which estimate risks by combining the results of several different studies, have drawn differing conclusions: two conclude that long-term use does not increase risk, one suggests that the risk may be elevated in naturally menopausal women, and one suggests that a 30 per cent increase in risk might be expected after fifteen years of oestrogen use (see Brinton and Schairer, 1993).

Conclusive data on the effects of long term *opposed* use are also sadly lacking. A study published in the early 1980s (Gambrell, 1983) which suggested that taking oestrogens with progestogens as HRT gave substantial protection from breast cancer was widely, and often uncritically, quoted. This hypothesis has yet to be supported; indeed, the few substantial studies with any data on opposed therapy which have been published subsequently suggest that the risk of combined therapy may even be higher (Ewertz, 1988; Bergkvist *et al.*, 1989; Kaufman *et al.*, 1991; Palmer *et al.*, 1991).

Despite the efforts of researchers, uncertainties about these two crucial questions are unlikely to be resolved in the immediate future; definitive data will only be available when the treatments have been used for substantial periods of time. This is clearly of little comfort to women who are currently using, or contemplating using, HRT.

Cardiovascular Disease

With the concerns expressed about both endometrial and breast cancer, it is likely that HRT would have remained as a form of therapy which was used short-term to alleviate vasomotor (and associated) symptoms by the minority of women who are incapacitated by such symptoms, and long-term by the minority of women who had been identified as being at high risk of early bone loss and osteoporosis. However, the publication throughout the 1980s of numerous papers which suggested a substantial protection from coronary heart disease has been crucial in reactivating calls for widespread long-term preventive use of HRT for the majority of post-menopausal women.

The first study to provide a convincing suggestion of a potential cardioprotective effect of unopposed HRT was published in 1981 and reported that the risk of ischaemic heart disease amongst recent users of oestrogens was less than half that for other women (Ross *et al.*, 1981). Several studies since then have also reported lower rates of heart disease in users of unopposed oestrogens (see Hunt and Vessey, 1991a; Meade and Berra, 1992). Whilst this substantial lowering of such a common form of illness and mortality is encouraging for users of HRT, it is important to note that it is not yet known whether taking progestogens together with oestrogens will take away this apparent cardioprotection. Meade and Berra summarise the current picture thus:

> 'the cardiovascular effects of progestogens used with oestrogen in ... women who have not undergone hysterectomy are unknown ... [T]he effects of different formulations on cardiovascular disease constitute one of the most pressing but complex issues in present-day medical practice' (Meade and Berra, 1992, p. 276).

Patterns of Prescribing HRT

Given the changing evidence on adverse and beneficial consequences of HRT use, it is perhaps not surprising that numbers of prescriptions for HRT have oscillated wildly. During the first half of the 1970s, prescriptions for hormonal preparations issued for treatment of menopausal symptoms rose steadily in the UK, reaching a peak between 1976 and 1977 when prescription figures were almost two and a half times as great as in 1972. Until 1975, these figures were virtually exclusively for unopposed HRT. The prevalence of use of HRT fell by around 30 per cent between 1977 and 1980 in response to publicity about the increased risk of endometrial cancer, and the overall figures remained steady through the early and mid-1980s (although the proportion of the total taken up by opposed therapy rose steadily during the decade from 1975 to 1985) (see Hunt and Vessey, 1987) as opposed therapy gradually became the norm for women who had not had a hysterectomy.

By 1985, much was in place for the rehabilitation of HRT; anxieties about endometrial cancer were fading in much of the medical and lay literature and data suggesting a large potential cardioprotective effect of unopposed HRT was accumulating. A second dramatic upsurge in the prevalence of use can be seen in the late 1980s and early 1990s.[3] Although the British Parliamentary Under-Secretary of State for Health stated recently that the 'number of prescriptions for [HRT] has quadrupled in the past decade' (Hansard Commons, 26 October 1993, column 683), in fact all of this increase took place in the five year period between 1987 and 1992. By 1992, the number of prescriptions for oestrogens and HRT in England was in excess of four and a half million, with a net ingredient cost of over £60 million (Hansard Commons, 26 October 1993, column 684; Department of Health, personal communication). In the mid-1970s, an editorial in *The Lancet* noted that longer term use of HRT to prevent osteoporosis would provide a lucrative market: 'the prospect of universal treatment of a large section of the female population is clearly a glittering prize for the pharmaceutical manufacturer' (*The Lancet*, editorial, 1975); this remains true in the 1990s, although the rationale for prevention is now broader, encompassing cardiovascular disease. The prospect of the use of HRT in the prevention of cardiovascular disease raises the question not only of medicalization of the menopause, but of the entire post-menopausal period. The establishment of such practice would indeed be a 'glittering prize', and would have widespread implications for the health service in addition, of course, for the lives and experiences of the women who were taking it.

Although epidemiological evidence on aspects of the long-term benefits and risks of HRT continues to accumulate, the epidemiological debate will remain unresolved for some years, even within the relatively narrow conceptions of benefits and risks as commonly defined. Most of the existing evidence is on the effects of long-term use of *unopposed* therapy, and inevitably there is debate and uncertainty about how the overall balance of effects will be altered by the use of progestogen-opposed treatment. This is further complicated by the fact that, increasingly since the early 1980s, women taking opposed HRT are those who have not had a prior hysterectomy, whilst those taking unopposed HRT are more commonly women who have had their uterus removed (often with the removal of one or both ovaries). The dynamic patterns of prescribing (both temporally and geographically) add an extra layer of complexity to the conduct and interpretation of epidemiological data. Women receiving HRT are likely to have been more or less carefully selected at different times and places: some studies may consist largely of healthier women with access to greater resources and lower intrinsic risk of the diseases which have featured prominently in the medical debate over HRT, whilst others may more closely resemble the general population (Hunt and Vessey, 1991a).

MacPherson has characterized the recent history of the use of HRT in relation to three 'false promises': the first phase, from 1966 to 1975, is characterized by the promise of eternal beauty and femininity; the second, from 1975 to 1981, by the promise of a safe, symptom-free menopause; and the third, 1980 to the present, by the promise of escape from chronic diseases (MacPherson, 1993). This characterization elegantly summarizes the debate in many ways, although in reality, elements of all three are often invoked in popular images of HRT and in promotional literature. Proclamations of the miraculous dual benefits of HRT as the elixir of 'youth' (as demonstrated largely by conformity to specific models of 'appropriate' femininity and sexuality) and as the cure for all major ills have been most prominent when sales of HRT have been climbing or about to climb (i.e. in the early 1970s, and the late 1980s and early 1990s) when the delicate balance between prophylaxis and adverse consequences has seemed to favour the 'benefits' side of the equation. A recent parliamentary question from Theresa Gorman could serve as an illustration:

> Given the amazing benefit from [HRT], of which I am an amazing example and the fact that this treatment could save the health service millions of pounds, because without it women are currently likely to suffer from osteoporosis, strokes[4] and other terrible diseases, does [the Parliamentary Under-Secretary of State for Health] not agree with me that the health service should be encouraged to dedicate funds so that lots more women can grow old gracefully?' (Hansard Commons, 26 October 1993, column 693).

Seldom have the promises of eternal beauty and femininity and fewer health problems remained separate, nor is reference to apparent cost-effectiveness and health service savings just a feature of the more consumerist, cost-conscious, post-reform NHS.

Medical and Popular Representations of Women as Reproductive Beings

The Menopause: Mid-life Passage, or the Beginning of the End?

Although the pursuit of 'male' and 'female' hormones dates back to the early twentieth century (see Vines, 1993, pp. 13–35 and Worcester and Whatley, 1992, pp. 41–44 for summaries), the 'promise' of HRT as a means of escaping the symptoms (and consequences) of the menopause only began to gain popular and medical currency in the 1960s. However, the construction of a 'menopausal syndrome' has neither been straightforward nor politically neutral. Although all women who have had periods have a definable menopause in the strict biological sense, namely the cessation of menstruation, the broader experience of the menopause (or climacteric), as the result of a complex interplay between bodily sensations and social and cultural expectations, is far from universal. Underlying the debate surrounding definitions of the menopause is a tension between the menopause as 'natural' and the menopause as 'pathological', and a looseness of language which reflects and perpetuates underlying aetiological ideologies. It is over half a century since Marie Stopes commented that:

> 'The change' and 'the critical period' for men and women are the popular equivalents of the scientific term *climacteric* used for the phase of evolution long widely recognised in women ... The menopause, however ... indicates a more limited and definite thing, the cessation of the menstrual flow of women. The menopause therefore may be complete itself while the climacteric continues, because other internal re-arrangements are going on during the climacteric (Stopes, 1950, p. 23).

That such ambiguities of language persist, despite the fact that most texts on the menopause since that time begin by trying to restrict the use of terms, reflects cultural ambiguities and the tension between medical and lay terminology.

Whilst the narrow definition of the 'menopause' seems relatively unproblematic (though has proved unsustainable), there is ambiguity even here, particularly since recent developments have heralded the possibilities of post-menopausal motherhood ('Menopause found no boundary to pregnancy', see Smith, 1993) and thus even the cessation of fertility, until recently the only universal marker of the menopause, seems more of a technicality than an inevitability. As Lock (1982) states, 'the occurrence of the actual menopause can only be assessed in retrospect after an interval of twelve months of complete amenorrhea which adds to the ambiguity, and possibly accounts for the universal lack of ritual associated with the biological event' (Lock, 1982, p. 264).

Studies conducted within the 'developed' Western world reveal little consensus about which symptoms may constitute a 'menopausal syndrome' and problems of studying 'the menopause' have been well documented (see, for example, McKinlay and Jefferys, 1974; Bungay,

1979; and Kaufert and Syrotuik, 1981). As Kaufert and Syrotuik have pointed out:

> Symptom lists range in length from one item to more than thirty. The symptoms in a list may be undifferentiated as in the Blatt index (Blatt, 1953) or grouped into sub-categories labelled 'psychological', 'psychosomatic', 'vasomotor' and/or 'somatic'. The classification of such symptoms is not even consistent between these lists: for example, 'palpitations' are categorized as psychological by Greene (1976), psychosomatic by Neugarten (1965), and vasomotor in the International Health Foundation Index (1977) (Kaufert and Syrotuik, 1981, p. 173).

Many studies (and lay images) are dominated by the experience of clinical populations (although clinic populations are atypical of the general population in several respects [see, for example, Ballinger, 1985; Hunt, 1988]) and until recently few data were available about the general experience of the menopause. In addition to individual weaknesses of earlier studies, Bungay (1979) noted that they share a number of problems: they are often cross-sectional (although longitudinal inferences are commonly drawn); they often rely on retrospective recall with all its inherent biases; and response-biases are introduced by being clearly about 'the menopause'. As Kaufert and Syrotuik remark:

> In menstrual and menopause research, there is a risk that stereotypes will become operative whenever the subjects of the research are aware of the topic of the research. Bias [becomes] a possibility regardless of whether they are reporting a present or past symptomatology (Kaufert and Syrotuik, 1981, p. 177).

Cross-cultural work reinforces the fallacy of a universal 'menopausal syndrome' and has raised doubts even about vasomotor symptoms. Townsend and Carbone (1980), in their review of earlier anthropological literature, have demonstrated wide variation in presentations of the menopause. Drawing on the work of Griffin (1977) and others, they report that 'apparently, in few of the world's cultures is there report of changed behaviour', although they do report evidence for 'withdrawal from social behaviour', 'greater freedom and privilege' and the gaining of 'specific supernatural and social powers' in others (Townsend and Carbone, 1980, p. 231). However, these observations are based on studies where the menopause was seldom the focus of research, reflecting the tradition in classical anthropology:

that women may not have been given the kind of attention by anthropologists which is their due as half of most populations partly because their own societies, and also the world of academic social anthropology, have viewed them under the influence of dominant male systems of perceptions (Ardener, 1977, p. xii).

In this sense, women have represented a 'muted group' (Ardener, 1977), and a paucity of data on many aspects of their lives and experiences has only begun to be redressed in the last twenty years.[5]

Data from anthropologists who have explicitly researched the menopause in 'other' cultures suggest very wide diversity. Flint suggests that, in contrast to the USA, reports of few problems at the menopause other than menstrual changes among Rajput women may result from the positive role changes ('rewards') resultant on becoming menopausal (Flint, 1975). Similar findings have been reported for older 'immigrant' Sikh women in British Columbia (George, 1988). Beyene, contrasting the menopausal experiences of Greek and Mayan women, however, concludes that 'cultural factors such as status gain and removal of taboos are inadequate explanations for variation in menopausal experiences' (Beyene, 1986, p. 67). Lock, in her extensive work on attitudes to the menopause in Japan, reports that there is no word in Japanese used specifically to describe hot flushes, and that the prevalence of the 'characteristic' somatic symptoms (hot flushes, night sweats and sudden perspirations) is low: 12.6 per cent and 10.8 per cent of peri- and post-menopausal Japanese women, respectively, reported hot flushes in the previous two weeks as compared with 39.7 per cent and 38.6 per cent of women from a comparable study in Manitoba (Lock, 1986). She concludes elsewhere that:

> despite the paucity of data, it is clear that there is enormous variation and that only the cessation of menses and decreased estrogen production are universal events, while hot flushes and sweats probably occur in most cultures but are by no means inevitable and are not necessarily associated with the menopause... The experience is subject to considerable social and cultural conditioning (Lock, 1982, p. 264).

Given this background, it is not surprising that there are competing constructions of the menopause, nor that some provide more obvious rationales (and markets) for HRT than others. A number of writers (see, for example, Lock, 1982; Kaufert, 1982; Kaufert and Gilbert, 1986; Bell,

1987) have contrasted biomedical and socio-cultural presentations of the menopause. Kaufert, for example, examined 'two competing descriptions of menopausal experience, one proffered by the medical profession and the other by the women's health movement [which are treated as "myths"]... that is, as systems of values which are presented as systems of fact, and therefore necessarily involve some distortion' (Kaufert, 1982, p. 141).

Recent work has supplemented earlier analyses. Dickson (1993) identifies 'four scientific paradigms of menopausal research with differing foundational assumptions...: the biomedical, the socio-cultural, a feminist, and a postmodern'. Zita (1993) describes three 'rhetorical strategies': biological essentialism ('menopause as the loss of true femininity'), scientific reductionism ('menopause as dysfunctional or functionless state'), and feminist valorization ('menopause as a "natural" life event'). The first two locate the menopause as a 'situation in the body, caused by internal dysfunction' and as such construe the menopause as negative, universal, sex-linked and 'siphoned off from cultural, historical and social contexts' (p. 64). In biological essentialist views, woman 'both *is* her biology and is determined by her biology. Menopause is perceived as an estrogen-deficiency disease, a deviation from the norms of true femininity' (p. 62) and as 'a deviance in gender ontology requiring medical intervention', and it converts a woman into a 'neuter' or non-woman. In scientific reductionist models, menopause is viewed as deviation from the norms of health and internal well-functioning (rather than gender *per se*) and is again portrayed as a dysfunctional state requiring medical intervention (usually HRT) and medical expertise and authority. The key features of the 'feminist valorization' of the menopause are that the menopause is a 'natural' rather than pathological life transition, which is variously experienced, and thus requires a range of interventions or no intervention depending on the ease or difficulty of individual experience. 'The body is a bio-cultural text; in part biologically given and in part culturally constructed ... [It] is "naturalized" by its relationship to a woman's entire life cycle' (p. 68) and is a personal, physical, cultural, and political event.

There is, of course, a diversity in both medical (see, for example, Lock, 1985; Wilkes and Meade, 1991) and feminist opinions about HRT and the menopause. As Lewis (1993) has remarked:

the HRT debate is particularly complicated in terms of the positions adopted by the actors participating in it: the medical profession has not spoken with a single voice and nor have lay (chiefly women) popularizers, while there is a significant body of epidemiological and social-science research which takes a very different tack from the clinical literature...there is no one feminist view of the menopause any more than there is one feminism. But the feminist literature tends to be universally suspicious of HRT (Lewis, 1993, pp. 38 and 50).

And she adds that, 'in many respects, the divisions in the specialist literature on HRT are made worse by the fact that they are rarely acknowledged to exist' (Lewis, 1993, p. 47).

Although the different models have quite different agendas and lend themselves to huge variations in potential size of 'market' for HRT, they have, on occasions, invoked similar concerns when eliciting support. On the basis of her analysis of examples of a medical and a feminist text on the menopause, Kaufert has pointed out that both the 'medical' and 'feminist' presentations of the menopause have exploited a fear of cancer 'to promote or demote medical control over the menopause experience' (Kaufert, 1982, p. 153). According to the medical view which she examines, women who choose not to consult a doctor when they experience irregular menses (and thereby take the responsibility of diagnosing the menopause themselves) may 'risk' failing to detect underlying pathology, and thus forego the benefits of early detection and treatment. In the 'feminist' view (as represented by material from the National Women's Health Network) women are warned that the presentation of 'menopausal' symptomatology may lead to risks of iatrogenic cancers.

It is not, of course, just images of cancer, but also of other aspects of ill-health and chronic illness or disability that are used, both in marketing material aimed at medical practitioners and in popular 'information' on HRT. Worcester and Whatley remark that 'the marketing of hormone products to menopausal and post-menopausal women is particularly cruel in the way that it plays on the fears of specific disabling or life-threatening conditions and also, very purposefully, on women's fear of ageing' (Worcester and Whatley, 1992, p. 3).

Kate Hunt

A Bloody Mess? Similarities Between Constructions of the Menopause and of Menstruation, Hormonal Cyclicity and the 'Essence' of Femininity

A striking feature of constructions of the menopause is their similarity to constructions of other aspects of female 'biology': they are the embodiment of the pervasive tendency to dichotomize 'male' from 'female' and rigidly proscribe their 'characteristics'. Recourse to models of sickness, ill-health and organic dysfunction are intimately linked to constructions of 'appropriate' and 'inappropriate' femininity and the enactment of female roles as documented (both historically and contemporaneously) in relation to hysteria (see Smith-Rosenberg, 1974), PMT (see Laws, 1983), and medical treatment of women more generally (see Ehrenreich and English, 1979; Scully and Bart, 1981). As Laws says of Katharina Dalton, the proponent of PMT:

> she is a defender of the ideal of the traditionally feminine woman. She gives statistics which blame women for a most extraordinary range of acts of disruptive violence, yet maintains at the same time that women are innocent, misunderstood victims of their hormones...Her patients want to be *nice*...[and] so far as judges are concerned *women* are never violent, aggressive, anti-social, women with PMT are (Laws, 1983, p. 21, emphasis in original).

Examples of the 'consequences' of the menopause for femininity are prolific; the following example comes from Cooper's *No Change*. After asserting that in the past the main meaning of the menopause was the 'relief from the annual ordeal of childbirth', she continues:

> The train of events that followed, the adverse effects on energy, health and appearance, were simply accepted as an inevitable part of ageing. Nature clearly lost interest in the infertile woman and saw no purpose in keeping her desirable...Alongside the compensation of being free of childbearing, a woman who survived beyond midlife had to accept that she was old and had ceased to be sexually interesting. The menopause marked the end of her life as a desirable woman, and, since she could no longer produce sons, it also reduced her value as a wife (Cooper, 1983, p. 64).

Wilson's notorious *Feminine Forever*, as its title suggests, is replete with further examples.

Menopause, menstruation (Laws, 1990), pregnancy, childbirth, are all convenient female hormonal 'states' on which to pin evidence of female inferiority. Together they span most of the life course. 'Problems' with any of these 'natural' processes (including constitutive experiences such as the pain associated with childbirth or menstruation) are taken as signs of the rejection of 'proper' female roles.

Countless illustrations abound in relation to the menopause. The following quote from a BMA booklet contains in its triteness and superficialities a succinct allusion to most of the supposed 'female' characteristics which can 'protect' against menopausal problems if properly deployed:

> I must have known [my grandmother-in-law][6] throughout her menopause; but she didn't know that she had had it until in her early fifties she suddenly remembered that she hadn't had a period for two years. What is her secret? I think probably in the first place she never nibbled between meals; in the second place that she had always been interested in other people; in the third place that she had always been a good dancer; in the fourth place that she had to look after her home and care for two husbands in succession; and last but not least that she has seen to it that she has stayed attractive enough for them to care for her in *every* possible way. She made herself an indispensible support for those around instead of demanding support from those around (Phillip, undated, p. 15).

The proper observance of designated moral standards to protect against ill-health, whilst often directed at women, is of course a pervasive theme in many aspects of health and disease (see for example, Crawford, 1985; Sontag, 1978, 1991).

A second similarity is the scant disregard for the lack of evidence to support the hormonal basis for female 'troubles' or female behaviour, and the tendency to extrapolate from clinical perceptions of clinical populations to presumed general experience. Thus, the common clinical impression that menopausal women are prone to psychiatric disorders, especially depression, persists although there is 'no clear research evidence' (Osborn, 1984, p. 126) for a link between depression and endo-crinological changes subsequent to the menopause *per se* (McKinlay *et al.*, 1987).[7] In relation to premenstrual syndrome (PMS) Golub has noted that, according to the definition in Webster's New Collegiate Dictionary of a syndrome (a 'group of signs and symptoms that occur together and characterize a particular abnormality'), 'premenstrual syndrome does not exist. To date no abnormality has been found, though many have been postulated' (Golub, 1992, p. 181; see also Vines, 1993). It does indeed seem that

> a little thing like lack of evidence does not make the least difference in the face of the widely-held male belief that women's behaviour is determined by 'raging hormonal influences'. Everyone *knows* that women who are violent, upset, unfeminine etc., have imbalanced hormones anyway... The root, of course, is femaleness, flawed femaleness (Laws, 1983, p. 29).

The third obvious similarity concerns issues of medicalization and medical control which rely simultaneously on the dichotomization between natural and pathological, but yet ensure that the two can never be 'safely' distinguished. Many previous authors have challenged medicalization of aspects of 'normal' life, notably in relation to pregnancy and childbirth (see, for example, Oakley, 1980) and medical texts have provided a rich source of evidence of the pathologization of the normal (see Smith-Rosenberg, 1974; Ehrenreich and English, 1979; U205 course team, 1985; Martin, 1989; and Barbre, 1993 as examples). Where medical uncertainty coexists with medicalization and medical control the debate is particularly charged. Awareness of this uncomfortable juxtaposition in an increasingly litigation-conscious era may explain part of the prevalent tendency to stress the need to involve women in (the responsibility for) decision-making about the use of HRT.

A fourth similarity is the importance and influence of individuals (both 'expert' and lay) as advocates for 'syndromes' and therapies. Robert A. Wilson is perhaps the most infamous of the North-American advocates who view the menopause and post-menopause as a pathological state of oestrogen-deficiency. His dramatic use of language leaves no room for doubt that life beyond forty-five or so is a wholly negative experience for women: 'no woman can be sure of escaping the horror of this living decay' (Wilson, 1966, p. 43). Only with HRT is the menopause curable and preventable; 'instead of being condemned to witness the death of their own womanhood... [women] will remain fully feminine — physically and emotionally — for as long as they live' (Wilson, 1966, quoted in Barbre, 1993, p. 32). A full thirty years after the publication of *Feminine Forever*, no fewer than seven of eleven chapters in a recent collection make explicit reference to his views (see Callahan, 1993).

In Britain, Cooper's *No Change* (which the author herself says 'could never be an uncommitted book' [p. 11]) has fulfilled a similar role in the 1970s and 1980s. Although Cooper describes herself

> as a woman [writing] for other women ... almost ten years later in the age of Women's Liberation, my approach is less romantic[8] and more rational [than Wilson's], with perhaps less emphasis on femininity and more on feminism, and the right of women to more say in decisions medical or social which affect their own bodies and their own lives (p. 19).

much of the essence of her analysis is very similar:

> It is the duty of modern medicine to ensure that the extra years [of life] that it has won for [women] are lived comfortably and fully, not crippled and limited by the effects of oestrogen deficiency ... What can't be cured must be endured, and in the past women did just that. Now for the first time in history, where the menopause is concerned, they do not have to (pp. 12–13).

Her book contains numerous personal testimonies throughout (including her own and that of Wilson's wife).

The importance of such advocates in generating interest in and a wider market for HRT is reflected both in prescribing figures and research participants' own accounts. Amongst several thousand women recruited from menopause clinics in Britain during the 1970s and early 1980s, for example, fewer than a quarter claimed that they had never read anything about HRT, and a quarter specifically said that they had read *No Change*. One, typically, said: 'My GP did not recommend HRT. I had read and heard about it from various sources, mostly from the journalist Wendy Cooper ... I have recommended HRT to a great many women because of my own experience' (Hunt, 1988). Many women described how they had fought the system (in the days before consumerism in the NHS), and defied or challenged medical opinion to obtain treatment in ways which closely mirror Cooper's descriptions (e.g., Cooper, 1983, p. 81). Several authors (Laws, 1983; Golub, 1992; Vines, 1993) have documented the influential role played by Dalton as the advocate for the recognition of PMS as a disease, and the implications of its inclusion as psychopathology (Caplan *et al.*, 1992).

Dilemmas and Double Binds?

The use of HRT to 'cure' or prevent symptoms and consequences of the menopause is an important area for feminist debate, although not one where it is straightforward to formulate a single feminist perspective (see also Lewis, 1993; Vines, 1993, pp. 139–141). On the one hand, whilst there remain uncertainties about the balance of benefits and risks either at the individual or a public health level, both the epidemiological evidence and personal testimonies do suggest that the judicious use of HRT has a potentially important role. On the other hand, given that much of the history of the treatment of women in medicine (Ehrenreich and English, 1979) places emphasis on the 'myth of female frailty' and has the tendency to relate this to 'women's hazardous menstrual and reproductive cycles' (Clarke, 1983, p. 64), feminist literature must continue to be at least sceptical about HRT, if not 'universally suspicious' (Lewis, 1993).

Hence, the changing fortunes of HRT have widespread implications, beyond the lives and health of increasing numbers of individual women who survive to enjoy a substantial part of their lifespan beyond the menopause, for health care providers, for the pharmaceutical industry (where these changing fortunes represent the loss or gain of monetary 'fortunes'), and for the images of femininity which feed back into social constructions of gender.

Kowlowski has noted that 'our [North American] society seems to demand a distinct, preferably exaggerated transition for women from "youth" to "maturity" (read "obsolescence")' (Kowlowski, 1993, p. 3), catapulting the menopausal woman 'beyond the bounds of acceptable femininity, sexuality and appeal to masculine desire' (Harding, 1988/9, p. 39). Or, as Russell has noted, middle age (of which the menopause is an important cultural marker) 'marks the point at which women cease to be "relevant" as women and start instead to become simply old' (Russell, 1987, p. 125). Despite the fact that few transitions in the lifespan are so abrupt, ours is a society which appears uncomfortable with ambiguity and invests much in the maintenance of binary oppositions (young vs old, male vs female and masculine vs feminine [see Bem, 1993] and so on).

Thus, embodied within its very name, 'hormone replacement therapy', are powerful social messages. Vines has noted that:

> Hormones have now become part of our day-to-day language, a
> way of accounting for our own and other people's

behaviour . . . The very word 'hormone' implies reckless action . . . Both the controversy surrounding hormones and behaviour, and the persistence with which a link is sought, suggest the impact of powerful cultural imperatives. The fact that hormones are most often seen as 'something women have' is . . . most revealing of all (Vines, 1993, pp. 1 and 2).

The notion of 'replacement' emphasises that, in passing through the menopause, a woman has reached a stage of need, of loss, of deficiency; implicitly or explicitly in 'marketing' material (whether this is advertisements from the pharmaceutical industry or 'information' about the menopause in the lay media) it is not only her hormones that need to be restored but her gender, her womanhood, the essence of her femininity. Portrayals of the post-menopausal woman without HRT emphasise what 'proper' or 'desirable' femininity is by showing what women are like when they no longer have it. They are no longer youthful, attractive, sexually interesting (to men), they have lost their fertility and with it their 'purpose' (their ability to bring new life and to care for others). HRT offers redemption, the ability to defy the clock, to become the sort of picture of youthful femininity which is to be marvelled at, the focus of the 'does she, doesn't she?' speculation that frequently accompanies media features on HRT (see for example, Sadgrove, 1990). As with other aspects of gender 'management' (see West and Zimmerman, 1991) being the 'proper' sort of post-menopausal woman requires constant vigilance, if a fall into the undesirable ('natural') state is to be avoided.

Such images are relevant for women of all ages and are omnipresent; the 'double standard of ageing' permeates everywhere. In her analysis of the plight of actresses over fifty, Kowlowski describes film as

an insidiously powerful tool for telling us what we aren't as women and what we should be [and as the] annihilation of self-esteem that comes to us . . . in the form of entertain-ment . . . [C]onditioned for shame about our bodies as they age, we watch portraits of once-vital women degenerate before our eyes while the men they support, each his own Dorian Gray, retain supernatural youthfulness (Kowlowski, 1993, p. 7).

Or as Russell has commented:

The clichéd emphasis in our society on youth and physical attractiveness is a much more powerful oppressor — at all ages

— of women than of men. Whereas a man's desirability as a sexual and social being is often defined in terms of personality, intelligence, . . . success and earning capacity, a woman's is more closely circumscribed by her physical appearance . . . For women there are no redeeming cultural stereotypes for wrinkles, crows feet and bulges in the wrong places . . . All women are affected by the double standard, old women more cruelly so (Russell, 1987, pp. 127 and 130).

Just in case women manage to divorce such negative views of older women from the menopause, the language in medical discourses of the menopause is, typically, exclusively negative (as it is for other aspects of reproduction, see, for example, Golub, 1992, pp. 4–7; Laws, 1990), a tendency which many self-help books challenge even in their titles (e.g. Reitz, 1981; Hunter, 1990). Ovaries 'wither', 'atrophy', 'regress', even the healthy post-menopausal woman may be described as 'sex-steroid deficient' or as a 'castrate' (Martin, 1989; Dickson, 1993). The message is clear that normality and pathology cannot easily be distinguished in the post-menopause. As with menstruation in the reproductively active part of our lives (Laws, 1990), peri- and immediately post-menopausal women continue to live with the dual pressures of secrecy and scrutiny which centre on the state of their body as a reproductive entity. As Frank has remarked, although 'people construct and use their bodies . . . they do not use them in conditions of their own choosing, and their constructions are overlaid with ideologies' (Frank, 1991, p. 47). Even when we no longer menstruate ourselves, we continue to contend with the legacy of society's attitudes towards menstruation and the female body more generally. As Zita concludes:

'the body' is an organic entity with structures and functions which can break down and go awry; but it is also an object which acquires social meaning and social location through cultural practices, which in turn can profoundly affect the body's health, well-being and our lived interpretation of our own bodies (Zita, 1993, p. 75).

As constructions of masculinity and femininity relate closely to the shape, size, conduct and functioning of the physical body, presentations of the menopause (the transition between a body with reproductive potential to one without) and treatments for the menopause are a rich source of evidence for the construction of gender overall.

Notes

1 Many other dichotomies are emphasized in the construction of the menopause. As Rips (1993, p. 82) has remarked, 'through the study of menopause as a social construct, we can question the dichotomies that have importance in our society. The topic highlights the oppositions between female and male, old and young, reproductive and postreproductive, abnormal or pathological and healthy.'

2 The addition of a progestogen on a cyclical basis usually leads to a 'withdrawal bleed'. Evidence suggesting that this decreases the acceptability of long-term use of opposed HRT amongst some women (particularly those who view the cessation of menstruation as a positive bonus of the menopause) has led to the search for other regimens, such as low-dose continuous progestogen, which aim to eliminate 'withdrawal bleeding'.

3 Such dramatic fluctuations in the use of HRT are not confined to Britain but have been mirrored elsewhere. For example, sales of HRT in Sweden increased between 1973 and 1977 from 3.65 defined daily doses per thousand women to 11.8, and thereafter declined to 9.3 in 1980 (Persson *et al.*, 1983). In the USA where HRT has generally been most widely used, the number of non-contraceptive oestrogen containing retail prescriptions rose from 1966 to reach a 1970s peak of 28 million prescriptions in 1975. Sales of HRT declined slightly earlier, falling steadily between 1975 and 1979 to levels below those of 1966. A clear recovery in sales was already apparent in the USA between 1979 and 1983 (Kennedy *et al.*, 1985). Worcester and Whatley (1992) quote sources which indicate that oestrogen prescriptions jumped in the USA from 15 million prescriptions per year in 1979/80 to nearly 32 million in 1989, when the annual sales of Premarin alone were valued at $400 million and were expected to exceed $1 billion by 1995 (see Worcester and Whatley, 1992, p. 4).

4 Although many papers have reported on cardiovascular disease, the majority have looked at ischaemic heart disease, whilst the evidence is still relatively limited on cerebrovascular disease.

5 Such gender-blindness is not of course confined to this aspect of contemporary or classical social science, as many previous authors have pointed out.

6 This is a variation of the common tendency amongst male doctors to use the personal experience of a female relative to illustrate their faith in a procedure or therapy or to justify a particular stance. Wendy Cooper tells us that one of the women she had met who had been on HRT for over twenty years was 'Robert Wilson's own wife, Thelma. It is always a good test of a doctor's faith in his own treatment if he uses it on his own family, and this pioneer of HRT was certainly not afraid to prescribe [it] for his own wife in the very early days when it was still highly controversial medicine' (Cooper, 1983, p. 83).

7 Laws notes that the 'symptoms' of PMT which receive most concern are depression, anxiety and other aspects of mental health which 'do not "fit" with women's culturally-created notions of themselves as nice, kind, gentle etc. "Mood change" as such is often described as a symptom — demonstrating that change *as such* is not culturally acceptable' (Laws, 1983, p. 24).

8 Some statements belie this 'lack of romanticism': 'In many ways oestrogen has a place in the life of a woman rather like that of love itself. She is born with both, and both assume their greatest importance in her fertile years. What is more she may take them both very much for granted, and only fully realizes their value when they are gone' (p. 29).

References

ARDENER, S. (Ed.) (1977) *Perceiving Women*, First paperback edition (First published, 1975). London, Dent.

BALLINGER, S. E. (1985) 'Psychosocial stress and symptoms of menopause: a comparative study of menopause clinic patients and non-patients', *Maturitas*, **7**, 315–327.

BARBRE, J. W. (1993) 'Meno-Boomers and Moral Guardians: an exploration of the cultural construction of the menopause', in CALLAHAN, J. (Ed.) *Menopause. A Midlife Passage*, Bloomington and Indianapolis, Indiana University Press, pp. 23–35.

BELL, S. E. (1987) Changing ideas: the medicalization of the menopause, *Social Science and Medicine*, **24**, 535–542.

BEM, (1993) *The Lenses of Gender, Transforming the Debate on Sexual Inequality*, New Haven, Yale University Press.

BERGKVIST, L., ADAMI, H-O., PERSSON, I., HOOVER, R. and SCHAIRER, C. (1989) 'The risk of breast cancer after estrogen and estrogen-progestin replacement', *New England Journal of Medicine*, **321**, 293–297.

BEYENE, Y. (1986) 'Cultural significance and physiological manifestations of menopause. A biocultural analysis', *Culture, Medicine and Psychiatry*, **10**, 47–71.

BIRKE, L. I. A. and VINES, G. (1987) 'Beyond nature versus nurture: process and biology in the development of gender', *Women's Studies International Forum*, **10**, 555–570.

BOYLE, M. (1992) 'The abortion debate', in NICHOLSON, P. and USSHER, J. (Eds) *The Psychology of Women's Health and Health Care*, Basingstoke, Macmillan, pp. 124–151.

BRINTON, L. A. and SCHAIRER, C. (1993) 'Estrogen replacement therapy and breast cancer risk', *Epidemiologic Reviews*, **15**, 66–79.

BRINTON, L. A., HOOVER, R. and FRAUMENI, J. F. (1986) 'Menopausal oestrogens and breast cancer risk: an expanded case-control study', *British Journal of Cancer*, **54**, 825–832.

BUNGAY, G. (1979) 'A study of symptoms in middle life with special reference to the menopause', Oxford, MFCM part II Thesis.

CALLAHAN, J. C. (Ed.) (1993) *Menopause. A Midlife Passage*, Bloomington and Indianapolis, Indiana University Press.

CAPLAN, P. J., McCURDY-MYERS, J. and GANS, M. (1992) 'Should "premenstrual syndrome" be called a psychiatric abnormality?', *Feminism and Psychology*, **2**(1), 27–44.

CLARKE, J. N. (1983) 'Sexism, feminism and medicalism: a decade review of literature on gender and illness, *Sociology of Health & Illness*, **5**(1), 63–82.

COOPER, W. (1983) *No Change: A Biological Revolution for Women*, Second revised ed. London, Arrow.

CRAWFORD, R. (1985) 'A cultural account of "health": control, release, and the social body', in McKINLAY, J. B. (Ed.) *Issues in the Political Economy of Health Care*, UK edition, London, Tavistock Publications Ltd, pp. 60–103.

DICKSON, G. L. (1993) 'Metaphors of the menopause: the metalanguage of menopause research', in CALLAHAN, J. (Ed.) *Menopause. A Midlife Passage*, Bloomington and Indianapolis, Indiana University Press, pp. 36–58.

EHRENREICH, B. and ENGLISH, D. (1979) *For Her Own Good. 150 Years of Experts' Advice to Women*, London, Pluto Press (first published by Anchor/Doubleday, 1978).

EWERTZ, M. (1988) 'Influence of non-contraceptive exogenous and endogenous sex hormones on breast cancer risk in Denmark', *International Journal of Cancer*, **42**, 832–838.

FLINT, M. (1975) 'The menopause: reward or punishment?', *Psychosomatics*, **16**, 161–163.

FRANK, A.W. (1991) 'For a sociology of the body: an analytic review', in FEATHERSTONE, M., HEPWORTH, M. and TURNER, B.S. (Eds) *The Body: Social Processes and Cultural Theory*, London, Sage, pp. 36–102.

GAMBRELL, R.D., MAIER, R.C. and SANDERS, B.T. (1983) 'Decreased incidence of breast cancer in postmenopausal estrogen-progestogen users, *Obstetrics and Gynecology*, **62**, 435–443.

GEORGE, T. (1988) 'Menopause: some interpretations of the results of a study among a non-western group', *Maturitas*, **10**, 109–116.

GOLUB, S. (1992) *Periods. From Menarche to Menopause*, Newbury Park, Sage.

GRIFFIN, J. (1977) 'A cross-cultural investigation of behavioural changes at menopause, *Social Science Journal*, **14**, 49–55.

HARDING, J. (1988) 'Ageing, women and sexuality', *Radical Community Medicine*, **Winter 1988/9**, 37–43.

HUNT, K. (1988) 'Perceived value of treatment among a group of long-term users of hormone replacement therapy', *Journal of the Royal College of General Practitioners*, **38**, 389–401.

HUNT, K. and VESSEY, M. (1987) 'Long-term effects of postmenopausal hormone therapy', *British Journal of Hospital Medicine*, **November**, 450–460.

HUNT, K. and VESSEY, M. (1991a) 'The risks and benefits of hormone replacement therapy: an updated review', *Current Obstetrics and Gynaecology*, **1**, 21–27.

HUNT, K. and VESSEY, M. (1991b) 'Use of hormone replacement therapy and breast cancer risk', in SITRUK-WARE, R. and UTIAN, W.H. (Eds) *The Menopause and Hormonal Replacement Therapy. Facts and Controversies*, New York, Marcel Dekker, Inc, pp. 143–159.

HUNTER, M. (1990) *Your Menopause. Prepare Now for a Positive Future*, London, Pandora.

HUTCHINSON, T.A., POLANSKY, S.M. and FEINSTEIN, A.R. (1979) 'Post-menopausal oestrogens protect against fracture of the hip and distal radius: a case-control study', *The Lancet*, **ii**, 705–709.

JICK, H., WALKER, A.M. and ROTHMAN, K.J. (1980) 'The epidemic of endometrial cancer: a commentary', *American Journal of Public Health*, **70**, 264–267.

KAUFERT, P.A. (1982) 'Myth and the menopause', *Sociology of Health & Illness*, **4**, 141–166.

KAUFERT, P.A. and GILBERT, P. (1986) 'Women, menopause and medicalization', *Culture, Medicine and Psychiatry*, **10**, 7–21.

KAUFERT, P. and SYROTUIK, J. (1981) Symptom reporting at the menopause, *Social Science and Medicine*, **15**, 173–184.

KAUFMAN, D.W., PALMER, J.R., DE MOUSON, J., ROSENBERG, L., STOLLEY, P.D., WARSHAUER, M.E., ZAUBER, A.G. and SHAPIRO, S. (1991) 'Estrogen replacement therapy and the risk of breast cancer: results from the Case-Control Surveillance Study', *American Journal of Epidemiology*, **134**, 1375–1385.

KENNEDY, D.L., BAUM, C. and FORBES, M.B. (1985) 'Noncontraceptive estrogens and progestins: use patterns over time', *Obstetrics and Gynecology*, **65**, 441–446.

KITZINGER, S. (1992) *Ourselves as Mothers*, London, Dorling Kindersley.

KOWLOWSKI, J. (1993) 'Women, film, and midlife Sophie's choice: sink or Sousatzka?', in CALLAHAN, J.C. (Ed.) *Menopause. A Midlife Passage*, Bloomington and Indianapolis, Indiana University Press, pp. 3–22.

LAWS, S. (1983) 'The sexual politics of pre-menstrual tension', *Women's Studies International Forum*, **6**, 19–31.

LAWS, S. (1990) *Issues of Blood. The Politics of Menstruation*, London, Macmillan.

LEWIS, J. (1993) 'Feminism, the menopause and hormone replacement therapy', *Feminist Review*, **43**, 38–56.

LOCK, M. (1982) 'Models and practice in menopause: menopause as syndrome or life transition?', *Culture, Medicine and Psychiatry*, **6**, 261–280.

LOCK, M. (1985) 'Models and practice in medicine: menopause as syndrome or life transition?', in HAHN, R. A. and GAINES, A. D. (Eds) *Physicians of Western Medicine*, Dordrecht, D. Reidel Publishing Company, pp. 115–139.

LOCK, M. (1986) 'Ambiguities of aging: Japanese experience and perceptions of menopause', *Culture, Medicine and Psychiatry*, **10**, 23–46.

MACPHERSON, K. I. (1993) 'The false promises of Hormone Replacement Therapy and current dilemmas', in CALLAHAN, J. (Ed.) *Menopause. A Midlife Passage*, Bloomington and Indianapolis, Indiana University Press, pp. 145–159.

MARTIN, E. (1989) *The Woman in the Body: a Cultural Analysis of Reproduction*, Milton Keynes, Open University Press (first published by Beacon Press, 1987).

MCCREA, F. and MARKLE, G. (1984) 'The estrogen replacement controversy in the USA and the UK: Different answers to the same question?', *Social Studies of Science*, **14**, 1–26.

MCKINLAY, J. B., MCKINLAY, S. M. and BRAMBILLA, D. (1987) 'The relative contributions of endocrine changes and social circumstances to depression in mid-aged women', *Journal of Health and Social Behavior*, **28**, 345–363.

MCKINLAY, S. M. and JEFFREYS, M. (1974) 'The menopausal syndrome', *British Journal of Social and Preventive Medicine*, **28**, 108–115.

MEADE, T. W. and BERRA, A. (1992) 'Hormone replacement therapy and cardiovascular disease', *British Medical Bulletin*, **48**, 276–308.

OAKLEY, A. (1980) *Women Confined. Towards a Sociology of Childbirth*, Oxford, Martin Robertson & Co. Ltd.

OSBORN, M. (1984) 'Depression at the menopause', *British Journal of Hospital Medicine*, September, 126–129.

PAGANINI-HILL, A., ROSS, R. K., GERKINS, V. R., HENDERSON, B. E., ARTHUR, M. and MACK, T. M. (1981) 'A case-control study of menopausal estrogen therapy and hip fractures', *Annals of Internal Medicine*, **95**, 28–31.

PALMER, J. R., ROSENBERG, L., CLARKE, E. A., MILLER, D. R. and SHAPIRO, S. (1991) Breast cancer risk after estrogen replacement therapy: results from the Toronto Breast Cancer Study, *American Journal of Epidemiology*, **134**, 1386–1395.

PERSSON, I., ADAMI, H-O., LINDBERG, B. S., JOHANSSON, E. D. B. and MANELL, P. (1983) 'Practice and patterns of estrogen treatment in climacteric women in a Swedish population', *Acta Obstet Gynecol Scand*, **62**, 289–296.

PERSSON, I., ADAMI, H-O., BERGKVIST, L., LINDGREN, A., PETTERSSON, B., HOOVER, R. and SCHAIRER, C. (1989) 'Risk of endometrial cancer after treatment with oestrogens alone or in conjunction with progestogens: results of a prospective study', *British Medical Journal*, **298**, 147–151.

PHILLIP, E. (undated) *The Change*, A BMA booklet.

REITZ, R. (1981) *Menopause. A Positive Approach*, London, Unwin.

RIPS, J. (1993) 'Who needs a menopause policy?', in CALLAHAN, J. (Ed.) *Menopause. A Midlife Passage*, Bloomington and Indianapolis, Indiana University Press, pp. 79–91.

ROSS, R. K., PAGANINI-HILL, A., MACK, T. M., ARTHUR, M. and HENDERSON, B. E. (1981) 'Menopausal oestrogen therapy and protection from death from ischaemic heart disease', *The Lancet*, **i**, 858–860.

RUBIN, G. L., PETERSON, H. B., LEE, N. C., MAES, E. F., WINGO, P. A. and BECKER, S. (1990) 'Estrogen replacement therapy: remaining controversies', *American Journal of Obstetrics and Gynecology*, **162**, 148–154.

RUSSELL, C. (1987) 'Ageing as a feminist issue', *Women's Studies International Forum*, **10**, 125–132.

SADGROVE, J. (1990) 'HRT: Older women's friend or foe?', *The Guardian*, February 20th, 1990.

SCULLY, D. and BART, P. (1981) 'A funny thing happened on the way to the orifice: women in gynecology textbooks', in CONRAD, P. and KERN, R. (Eds) *The Sociology of Health and Illness*, New York, St. Martins Press.

SHAPIRO, S., KELLY, J.P., ROSENBERG, L., KAUFMAN, D.W., HELMRICH, S.P., ROSENSHEIN, N.B., LEWIS, J.L., KNAPP, R.C., STOLLEY, P.D. and SCHOTTENFELD, O. (1985) 'Risk of localized and widespread endometrial cancer in relation to recent discontinued use of conjugated estrogens', *New England Journal of Medicine*, **313**, 969–972.

SMITH, D.G., PRENTICE, R., THOMPSON, D.J. and HERMANN, W.L. (1975) 'Association of exogenous estrogen and endometrial carcinoma', *New England Journal of Medicine*, **293**, 1164–1167.

SMITH, P. (1993) 'Selfish genes and maternal myths: a look at postmenopausal pregnancy', in CALLAHAN, J. (Ed.) *Menopause. A Midlife Passage*, Bloomington and Indianapolis, Indiana University Press, pp. 92–119.

SMITH-ROSENBERG, C. (1974) 'Puberty to Menopause: the Cycle of Femininity in Nineteenth Century America', in HARTMAN, M. and BANNER, L.W. (Eds) *Clio's Consciousness Raised*, New York, Harper and Row, pp. 23–37.

SONTAG, S. (1989) *Illneess as Metaphor*, New York, Vintage.

SONTAG, S. (1991) *Illness as Metaphor and AIDS and its Metaphors*, London, Penguin.

STOPES, M.C. (1950) *Change of Life in Men and Women*, Fourth Edition (First published 1936) London, Putman and Co., Ltd.

TOWNSEND, J.M. and CARBONE, C.L. (1980) 'Menopausal syndrome: illness or social role — a transcultural analysis', *Culture, Medicine and Psychiatry*, **4**, 229–248.

U205 COURSE TEAM (1985) *Medical Knowledge: Doubt and Certainty*, Health and Disease Course, Book II. Milton Keynes, Open University Press.

VINES, G. (1993) *Raging Hormones. Do they rule our lives?* London, Virago.

WEISS, N.S., SZEKELY, D.R. and AUSTIN, D.F. (1976) 'Increasing incidence of endometrial cancer in the United States', *New England Journal of Medicine*, **294**, 1259–1261.

WEISS, N.S., URE, C.L., BALLARD, J.H., WILLIAMS, A.R. and DALING, J.R. (1980) 'Decreased risk of fractures of the hip and lower forearm with postmenopausal use of estrogen', *New England Journal of Medicine*, **303**, 1195–1198.

WEST, C. and ZIMMERMAN, D.H. (1991) 'Doing gender', in LORBER, J. and FARRELL, S.A. (Eds) *The Social Construction of Gender*, London, Sage, pp. 13–37.

WILKES, H.C. and MEADE, T.W. (1991) 'Hormone replacement therapy in general practice: a survey of doctors in the MRC's general practice research framework', *British Medical Journal*, **302**, 1317–1320.

WILKINSON, S. and KITZINGER, C. (1993) *Heterosexuality: A 'Feminism and Psychology' Reader*, London, Sage.

WILSON, R.A. (1966) *Feminine Forever*, New York, M. Evans.

WORCESTER, N. and WHATLEY, M.H. (1992) 'The selling of HRT: Playing on the fear factor', *Feminist Review*, **41**, 1–26.

ZIEL, H.K. and FINKLE, W.D. (1975) 'Increased risk of endometrial carcinoma among users of conjugated estrogens', *New England Journal of Medicine*, **293**, 1167–1170.

ZITA, J.N. (1993) 'Heresy in the female body: the rhetorics of menopause', in CALLAGHAN, J. (Ed.) *Menopause. A Midlife Passage*, Bloomington and Indianapolis, Indiana University Press, pp. 36–58.

Chapter 10

Widows' Weeds and Women's Needs: The Re-feminisation of Death, Dying and Bereavement

Jane Littlewood

This chapter is concerned with the health, both physical and psychological of widows in contemporary Britain. In many ways, the documentation of the experiences of widowhood which followed the Second World War stimulated the development of a whole body of research concerned with death, dying and bereavement. However, since the late 1970s, interest in widows as a specific group of bereaved individuals has been overtaken by the desire to broaden research concerning death-related issues into other areas of loss. Consequently, in a recent publication entitled 'Death, Dying and Bereavement' (Dickenson and Johnson, 1993), widows are not even referred to in the index despite widowhood being one of the numerically most frequent results of death. Nevertheless, the position of widows is in many ways unique, despite the processes associated with bereavement being similar across a range of losses. It will be argued here that factors affecting the grieving process amongst widows are, and always have been, inextricably linked to the consignment of women to the 'private' sphere, where they are conveniently forgotten, and to the domination of the 'public' sphere by men. It will further be suggested that post-war social policy provision for women who are widows operated actively to reinforce women's subordinate position in society. The 'Beveridge blueprint' for social policy in post-war Britain effectively defined women as the economic dependents of men in social and ideological terms whilst leaving them in practical terms, whether they worked outside of the home or not, severely under-insured in the event of their male partners' premature deaths.

My work in this area is located within the broader context of the de-medicalisation and associated re-feminisation of death, dying and bereavement. A growing body of work has already been produced concerning the acceleration of the medicalisation of these processes during the inter-war period. Furthermore, a substantial body of work concerning the re-feminisation, at least in terms of service provision, of the areas of death, dying and bereavement has also been produced. In contrast, little has been written concerning the experiences of widows, still less on lesbian 'widowhood', in contemporary society. Many widows alive today were widowed at a time when the masculinisation of death, dying and bereavement was at its peak.

The widows who are referred to in this chapter were interviewed in connection with work concerning adult reactions to bereavement in general (Littlewood, 1992a), and women's reactions to widowhood in particular (Littlewood, 1992b). Some widows were interviewed using a semi-structured interview schedule whilst others were members of the National Association of Widows who participated in a training day. Obviously, whilst the definition of widowhood is broadly based upon heterosexual marriage, the National Association of Widows turns no-one away. The semi-structured interview schedule was concerned with the following areas: social support, experience of bereavement, adjustment to loss and areas of particular difficulty. The first part of the training day was concerned with a discussion of the problems commonly experienced by widows and the second part of the day involved an in-depth discussion of two particular problems: i.e. the stigmatisation of widows and their sexuality.

The De-feminisation and Medicalisation of Death and Dying

Since the end of the nineteenth century in Europe there has been a revolution in traditional attitudes and feelings about death. Ariès (1975) has suggested that death has become shameful, hidden and forbidden. He further suggests that this change of attitudes was accelerated by the displacement of the site of death between 1930 and 1950. As Adams (1993) has indicated, this displacement of the social management of death effectively transferred control from the private, and largely feminine, sphere of the home to the public, and largely masculine, sphere of the hospital and the funeral director. Oakley (1979) makes a similar point when she suggests that the medical management of childbirth, childcare, dying and death changed 'from a structure of control located in a community of untrained women, to one based on a profession of formally trained men' (Oakley 1979, p. 18).

However, even within the realm of male scientific rationality women have continued to do the bulk of the often dirty and demanding emotional and physical work associated with caring for people who are dying (James, 1992). Consequently, this de-feminisation of the power to define and control the management of death was quickly challenged by women and alternatives to male, hospital based, technological approaches to terminal illness were sought.

The Re-feminisation of Death and Dying

As James and Field (1992) have pointed out, Cicely Saunders and Elizabeth Kübler-Ross, (the former being the founder of the modern hospice movement [1968] and the latter being the author of the highly influential book *On Death and Dying* [1969]) have effectively become charismatic leaders. Both women have revolutionised the care of people who are dying. However, as Walter (1993) indicates, the question of whether this transformation will succeed, or will be subverted, remains an open one. Alternatively, Adams (1993) has addressed the issues identified by Haggis (1990) regarding the under reporting of women's roles and rituals by identifying the central role played by working-class women in the inter-war years in the social management of death. However, Walter (1993) expresses surprise that feminists in particular have not paid greater attention to this area. Whilst he concedes the point that feminists have been concerned with the deaths of foetuses and infants, he asks whether challenging patriarchy in the care of people who are dying or who have been bereaved is seen as peripheral to the feminist task, since relatively little attention is paid to it. However, it may be argued that relatively little attention is paid to widows at all.

Widowhood as a Social Death

Three out of every four women who marry in Britain can expect to be widowed at some time in their lives. Whilst for most married women, widowhood will occur in the old age range, some will be bereaved in middle-age, typically by their partners suffering a terminal illness. A few will be widowed at a relatively young age, typically by their partners being involved in a fatal road traffic accident. Many women in the middle and younger age ranges will be left as the sole carers of young or teenaged children.

Mulkay (1993), in writing about death in general, makes some interesting observations concerning the social position of women in Victorian England — which has long been hailed by some, Geoffrey Gorer (1965) in particular, as a 'golden age' of grief. Gorer was particularly concerned about the position of widows following the Second World War. Specifically, he saw their social isolation increasing as a result of declining mourning customs in England. With the decline of mourning dress and the associated decline of the overt ritualisation of grief, he believed that social support for people who had been bereaved would inevitably decline, leaving widows in particular relatively isolated, unsupported, and prone to mental ill health.

Mulkay however, indirectly suggests the opposite: i.e. that widows, far from being the recipients of social support in Victorian England, were further removed from the public sphere following their husbands' deaths: 'the most lengthy and elaborate of all mourning sequences was that of a wife for a husband. Mourning dress of an exaggerated severity was worn for the first two years as a sign of "inner desolation". Black, light absorbing crèpe was used to express her grief and withdrawal from the world. For the first year of bereavement the widow could undertake no social activity outside of the home (Mulkay, 1993, p. 39). However, after the initial period of social withdrawal, Mulkay notes that one important function women did play in public life was representing, not themselves, but, at a time of relatively high mortality rates, the dead members of their family.

Morley (1971) and Walvin (1986) also note that working-class women took responsibility for mourning, as well as for the social management of death, by effectively keeping their dead 'alive' by means of regular prayers and visits to their graves. Mulkay is of the opinion that widowhood in contemporary society may be the start of what he terms 'the social death sequence' for women. Within the social death sequence, the woman who is no longer anyone's wife and who is no longer required to represent the dead within society, is politely required to disappear, preferably quietly.

Cochrane (1936), in a much earlier paper, identified a similar tendency and attempted to account for the social hostility towards, and avoidance of, widows. In a paper entitled 'A Little Widow is a Dangerous Thing,' he suggests that in many societies the social death, and in some instances the physical death, of women who had been widowed was commonplace. Parkes (1972) makes a similar point and argued that, at the time he was writing, widows in England were not burned but pitied and avoided instead.

Littlewood (1993a) suggests that these attitudes towards widows have persisted and may be related to the much higher levels of isolation and lower levels of social support widows report when compared to widowers. Furthermore, the profound sense of threat many women experience following the death of their husband may be directly related to the social circumstances in which they find themselves rather than in the individual woman's tendency towards neurosis. It is certainly the case that many widows are fully aware of a distinct social tendency to avoid women who have been widowed. Indeed, many keep their status hidden to avoid its negative connotations. For example, 'It's not something I reveal about myself on first acquaintance. It's a horrible word really, it conjures up Dickensian images of little women wearing black who should be pitied and patronised' and 'Music Hall jokes about merry and wise widows. Sexual connotations, dirty jokes, that sort of thing'; 'Husband stealers, that's what they call us.'

Alternatively, for some widows, their first experience of avoidance may come as a shock:

> I was still the same person but they crossed the road to avoid me. I could hardly believe they did that. They invited me out and when I got there, there was only one seat left at the table and John got up and got another chair. I spent the rest of the evening being ignored and sitting next to an empty chair.

Other widows are angry at the way they are treated: 'Society's attitude towards widows? I can tell you that one for nothing. It's piss off and die.'

The De-feminisation and Medicalisation of Bereavement

If the de-feminisation of the social management of death may be said to have accelerated from the 1930s onwards due to its relocation to the hospital from the community, then the de-feminisation of the management of bereavement was not far behind, and indeed bereavement was similarly medicalised. In a highly influential paper written in 1944, Lindemann referred to 'The Symptomatology and Management of Acute Grief', and by 1961, Engel was considering the question 'Is Grief a Disease?' However, the medical management of bereavement was essentially a psychiatric rather than a general medical enterprise.

During the late 1960s and early 1970s, stage/phase analyses were introduced, primarily by psychiatrists, in an attempt to explain the processes of dying and bereavement. For example, Averill (1968) identified shock, despair and recovery as the relevant stages of grief, and Kübler-Ross's (1969) analysis of the stages of dying (i.e. denial, anger, bargaining, depression and finally acceptance) was also applied to bereavement. In addition, Parkes (1972) identified numbness, pining, depression and recovery as the relevant stages which followed the loss of a loved person in adult life.

These stage/phase analyses of bereavement have been widely criticised. For example, Kastenbaum (1975) and Germain (1980) show how any theory which encourages the notion of one developmental path also implicitly encourages the labelling of any deviation from it as abnormal. Charmaz (1980) takes these criticisms further and argues that such theories do not necessarily reflect general patterns of coping but reflect adaptation to the particular social context in which the bereavement occurs. Littlewood (1993b) makes the further suggestion that stage/phase analyses of bereavement do not reflect the reality of grief at all. Rather, their attraction lies in their ability to represent experiences of bereavement in a manner suitable for the realm of male scientific rationality: i.e. as an experience which follows an ordered linear progression.

However, the experiences associated with grief are probably better characterised in terms of wave after wave of violently contradictory emotional impulses 'more of a cyclical thing really' and 'like waiting for the next wave to hit you'. Paradoxically, a stage/phase analysis of bereavement may make most sense to people who have never experienced the death of a close relative; i.e. in all probability the majority of young to middle-aged health care professionals. Indeed, such analyses were probably written *by* as well as *for* this group.

The De-feminisation of Widows

The experiences of widows have been central to the development of our understanding of bereavement. For example, the work of Marris (1958 and 1986) and Parkes (1972) was primarily concerned with widowhood. However, the fact that a widow is a woman seems to have been strangely overlooked. Consequently, our understanding of bereavement rapidly progressed into other areas without addressing key issues surrounding a widowed woman's needs. For example, Marris (1986) uses his previous research (Marris, 1958) concerning young-to-middle-aged widows as the cornerstone of his generic theory concerning loss and change. However, whilst he identifies the conventional lifestyles of women as being based upon economic and social dependence on men, he neither questions this arrangement nor speculates upon the specific impact that the death of a husband may have. Consequently, the work was generalised before it was properly understood.

He may be correct to point out that when a married man dies prematurely his wife's life may lose its meaning, but he fails to consider that this may be because the meaning of the women's life was specifically restricted to the private sphere of personal relationships. Furthermore, such restriction was not necessarily a matter of personal choice but it was certainly a matter of public policy. Consequently, he also fails to consider that a woman who is widowed loses considerably more than 'meaning' as she, often by necessity, enters the public sphere from a distinctly disadvantaged position. For example, 'I'd had no education, nothing to speak of, and I hadn't worked for years. It was hard, really hard'; and 'They didn't want women working then and I hadn't been to work since John was born'; and 'I don't know what I expected but I didn't expect to be that badly off.'

For many members of the National Association of Widows the Beveridge dream turned into a nightmare when their bereavement effectively plummeted them into poverty, stigmatisation and single parenting. For example:

> Well, I suppose I was a bit naive really. We kept ourselves to ourselves and I'd never had to claim social security but I found the whole thing to be offensive. It was sex from start to finish. It was the first time I realised how women were seen. Well, I mean my husband had just died and I felt raw and vulnerable I just wanted to scream at them.

and

> The thing I found most upsetting was losing my widow's pension when I re-married. Why? Oh, I suppose I felt it was a bit demeaning really . . . me and my kids being parcelled off from one man to another really.

Another recounted how:

> a friend of mine started to have a relationship with a man after her husband died and well, somebody reported her to the social and the upshot of it was that they tried to stop her widow's pension I mean the cheek of it — you don't stop being a widow

just because you start going out with somebody else — he wasn't prepared to keep her in any case.

The initial work of Parkes (1972) was also centrally concerned with the experiences of widows. This work was extended to include widowers by Glick *et al.* (1974), who reported that the overall differences between widows and widowers were small. However, they identified the following tendencies: widowers were more likely to attempt to control the expression of emotion, were more likely to report feeling themselves again at one year, were more likely to feel sexually deprived, and to think of re-marriage more quickly. The profound difficulties women in general, and widows in particular, experience in connection with the expression of their sexuality, not to mention the attempts of patriarchy to define and control it, were not discussed in any depth.

Also, Marris (1986) and Parkes (1972) both actively excluded elderly widows, i.e. the majority of widows, from their samples. Consequently, the problems faced by elderly widowed people, primarily isolation, loneliness and the prospect, in some cases, of admission to a residential or nursing home for elderly people have yet to be fully addressed. Due to the greater longevity of women, such problems may be expected to face considerably more women than men.

Overall, the experiences of widows have contributed a great deal to our understanding of bereavement without our understanding of bereavement contributing a great deal to our understanding of the specific problems faced by widows.

Experiences of Grief

The experiences associated with grief are many and varied and, in the case of widows, probably compounded by social isolation. In comparison to other groups of bereaved people widows tend to show higher levels of anxiety, hostility and anger. They also experience more loneliness and a greater sense of life's meaninglessness. However, complications can and do arise during the process of grief and one which frequently affects widows is that of chronic grief. However, there are also problems associated with physical health which frequently accompany the experience of bereavement.

As Osterweiss *et al.* (1984) have indicated, little is known about specific aspects of the biology of grief. However, in terms of the observations and experiences of bereaved people themselves, it would seem reasonable to suggest that respiratory, autonomic and endocrine systems may all be affected by phases of acute grieving. In addition, evidence from the epidemiology of bereavement would suggest that cardiovascular and immune function may be substantially altered by grief. Furthermore, the physiological effects of certain types of bereavement have been demonstrated in a number of studies. For example, Irvin *et al.* (1988) have demonstrated that natural killer cell activity, which is important to the body's defence against tumours and viral infections, is reduced in women undergoing conjugal bereavement.

Many studies have indicated that significant increases in mortality and morbidity follow the death of a loved person. Young *et al* (1963) found a major increase in the death rate of widowers aged fifty-four and over during the first six months following their bereavement, whilst Maddison and Viola (1968) found increased morbidity in widows. Kalish (1985) has suggested that such increases may be common following the death of any loved person and Rowland (1977) is of the opinion that the greatest risk of illness or death is during the first six months following bereavement.

In addition to these health risks, there are many other physical sensations associated with grief. The sensations most commonly reported are as follows:

1. Experiences of hollowness or tightness. Hollowness tends to be associated with the stomach or abdomen and tightness with the chest, shoulders and throat.
2. Over-sensitivity to noise.
3. A sense of depersonalisation.
4. Breathlessness, frequently accompanied by deep sighing respirations.
5. Muscular weakness.
6. Lack of energy and fatigue.
7. Dry mouth.

Although the physical sensations associated with grief may be experienced as frightening, they are not in themselves cause for concern.

The Grief of Widows

Anxiety, whilst common to all bereavements, may be particularly pronounced in widows. This anxiety can take many forms. Its most general manifestation is a pronounced fear of insanity. Many widows express the fear that the intensity of their grief will literally send them mad. Some widows suffer from a persistent sense of being unsafe in the world, whilst some experience panic attacks and agoraphobia.

Another source of anxiety, which is particularly pronounced in widows with children, is an increased awareness of one's own mortality. For example:

> I keep thinking something's going to happen to me, that I have cancer, or I'll be killed or something. The kids would be on their own then. I'm terrified of dying before they grow up. I keep thinking I might not live to see Amy's next birthday.

and

> Insurance, insurance. I spent most of my wages on insurance. I thought that at least they'd [her children] have some money if I died.

A final form of anxiety commonly reported by widows surrounds the issue of their sexuality. Jones (1988) comments at length upon her experience of her husband's terminal illness and death:

> I was more surprised to find how sexual is death. I now understand how a person whose partner is dying might, in some circumstances, go out and couple violently and casually. It would neither shock nor startle me, yet I might have lived all my life without this knowledge. Almost immediately Stanley went into hospital, I went out and bought new clothes; a pretty blouse, some knickers ... For a few days I went with the same high excitement I had felt when Stanley and I first met ... Somehow I knew I had felt all these things before, recognised them, but I never identified them until I was telling a young married woman of our acquaintance. She looked at me, tears in her eyes, and said 'Don't you know? You were courting!' And that was it. (Jones, 1988, p. 22)

Many widows are afraid of being perceived as sexually available, and some report instances of being sexually harassed by men of their acquaintance:

> Well, he just kept coming round to the house and saying he wanted to help and then he started coming when my daughter was at work, 'If you're ever desperate...' he says. I'd bloody well have to be I thought. Anyway, I threw him out.

and

> What? Oh, was anyone unhelpful to me? Well, there was this friend of Alan's, from work, I don't really want to go into the details but it was a sexual thing. I was absolutely terrified. I didn't go out of the house for a week.

Other widows felt ambivalent about their sexual needs and were unable to develop a strategy to defeat the combination of stigma, ageism and hostility they encountered. For example: 'Well, I mean I'm a mother aren't I and mums just don't do that sort of thing. Not when they've got adolescent kids at any rate.'; and 'My son was exceptionally difficult about it, "Mother, at your age!" he said.' Yet many women yearned for intimacy and felt quite unable to express their needs except perhaps in dreams of their dead husbands, which were common and frequently provoked anguish upon waking.

The anger and hostility expressed by widows is primarily targeted at a world perceived to be hostile to them and at the social isolation they feel they have little option but to endure. Avoidance and lack of social support from friendship networks also provoke anger in women who have been widowed. Many widows experience a pervasive and painful feeling that somehow they have been 'let down' by their husbands, their friends, or society in general. Given the social context in which many widows find themselves, it is their restraint, rather than their hostility, which is remarkable.

When complications arise during the grieving process of widows these are usually variants of chronic grief. For example, Gorer (1965) identified mummification, which involves a process in which the world of the bereaved person appears to be frozen in time following the death. The person who has been bereaved often behaves as if the dead person will return at some future date. Gorer cites Queen Victoria's reaction to the death of Prince Albert as an example of this form of chronic grief. However, it might be suggested that this example is potentially misleading since Queen Victoria, far from freezing her world in time, actively behaved as if Prince Albert was alive and interacting with her on a day to day basis. Marris (1986), in making a similar point regarding loss in general, cites a more accurate example of the form mummification may take. He uses an example from literature: Miss Haversham — a character in Dickens's *Great Expectations* who waited forever, in her tattered wedding gown, by the ruins of what should have been her marriage feast.

In very general terms, the mothers of children who have died, particularly when the death occurred in sudden and tragic circum-stances, are far more likely to behave in a manner similar to Miss Haversham than are widows. Arguably, such a response represents an attempt to avoid a psychological collapse, which may occur if the full impact of the loss is acknowledged.

Many widows, particularly elderly widows living alone in the community, behave in a manner reminiscent of Queen Victoria, i.e. they continue to behave as if their husbands were still alive. For example:

> Mrs B still thinks of her husband constantly and often talks to him as if he were still in the room with her. She points out things in the newspaper which she knows would interest him and watches TV programmes which she knows he would like (Littlewood, 1992a, pp. 113–114).

This pattern of reaction to bereavement amongst elderly people has now been so widely reported e.g. Raphael (1984) and Littlewood (1992a) that questions have been raised as to whether this reaction should be considered to be 'complicated' at all. It could well be the case that the exclusion of elderly respondents from the earlier work effectively masked a common response to loss amongst the older age ranges. Alternatively, this reaction may well be related to beliefs concerning an afterlife which are generally declining but still relatively common amongst older people. It could be the case that the next generation of elderly widows will react to their bereavement differently.

Another variation of chronic grief which is not unusual amongst widows is that of 'encapsulation'. Parkes (1975) identified encapsulation as a response to what he called redundant world models. Encapsulation involves effectively 'boxing off' an experience which threatens an individual's world view. For example, many widows still felt themselves to be the age they were when their husband died. Others used dreams as vehicles for encapsulation: 'I'm always forty-seven in dreams. The age I was when he died. The children are the same age as they were when he died too.' 'The dreams? Oh always happy dreams. Dreams of when we were together as a family.' Only 10 per cent of widows re-marry following the death of their partner. Whilst in many cases the longevity of women leads to a shortage of potential partners, equally many women make a conscious decision not to re-marry.

In many ways the complications arising from the grieving process amongst widows can be interpreted as an adaptation to the social position in which they find themselves. Maintaining a relationship with a dead partner may well be preferable to dying a social death.

Jane Littlewood

The Re-feminisation of Bereavement

The history of the medicalisation of bereavement has been as short as the history of the medicalisation of death. As Walter (1993) has indicated, the area of bereavement counselling has also produced a female charismatic leader (Torrie) and bereavement is now increasingly being dealt with by largely female counsellors, social workers, self-help groups and befrienders, as opposed to largely male members of the clergy and the psychiatric profession. Furthermore, bereavement is increasingly being seen as an inevitable part of life which requires a series of painful personal adjustments to be made, rather than as a form of psychiatric disturbance.

In many ways, the contribution of widows to our understanding of bereavement has been enormous. However, I have attempted to show that when, and increasingly if, a woman dons widows' weeds we forget that she has a woman's needs. Women widowed in post-war Britain were socialised into a patriarchal society at a particular time in history when certain roles for women were actively being prescribed. The impact of this on a woman's experience of widowhood coupled with society's attitude toward women should not be underestimated. Mulkay (1993) has expressed the hope that as the position of women in society changes then so will the position of widows.

Nevertheless, the experiences of widows during the post-war period of Britain are not wholly negative. These women have effectively developed strategies to overcome their disadvantaged position and many have deprived a potentially hostile society of the convenience of their social death.

In a difficult and painful situation, which is known to carry an increased risk of psychological and physical ill health, many have successfully combined a career with the sole parenting of their children. Others have actively campaigned to improve the financial and social position of widows. Theirs has been an essentially invisible task which has been achieved against all of the sociological odds. The widows of post-war Britain need neither pity nor avoidance. Rather, we should applaud them for their resilience and for their resistance.

References

ADAMS, S. (1993) 'A gendered history of the social management of death and dying in Foleshill, Coventry, during the inter-war years', in CLARK, D. (Ed.) *The Sociology of Death*, Oxford, Blackwell.

ARIÈS, P. (1975) *Western Attitudes Towards Death*, London, The John Hopkins University Press.

AVERILL, (1968) 'Grief: its nature and significance', *Psychological Bulletin*, **70**, 721–48.

CHARMAZ, K. (1980) *The Social Reality of Death*, Reading, Mass., Addison-Wesley.

COCHRANE, A. L. (1936) 'A little widow is a dangerous thing', *International Journal of Psycho-Analysis*, **17**, 494.

DICKENSON, D. and JOHNSON, M. (Eds) (1993) *Death, Dying and Bereavement*, London, Sage.

ENGEL, G. (1961) 'Is grief a disease?', *Psychosomatic Medicine*, **23**, 18–22.

GERMAIN, C. P. (1980) 'Nursing the dying: implications of the Kubler-Ross Staging Theory', in FOX, R. (Ed.) *The Social Meaning of Death, Annals of the American Academy of Political and Social Science*, **447**, 46–58.

GLICK, I. O., WEISS, R. S. and PARKES, C. (1974) *The First Year of Bereavement*, New York, Wiley.

GORER, G. (1965) *Death, Grief and Mourning in Contemporary Britain*, London, Cresset Press.

HAGGIS, J. (1990) 'The feminist research process', in STANLEY, L. (Ed.) *Feminist Praxis*, London, Routledge.

IRVIN, M., DANIELS, S., RISCH, C., BLOOM, E. and WEINER, H. (1988) 'Plasma cortisol and natural killer cell activity during bereavement.' *Biological Psychiatry*, **24**, 173–8.

JAMES, N (1992) 'Care = organisation + physical labour + emotional labour', *Sociological Review*, **37**, 15–42.

JAMES, N. and FIELD, D. (1992) 'The routinisation of hospice', *Social Science and Medicine*, **34**, 1363–75.

JONES, M. (1988) *Secret Flowers: Mourning and the Adaptation to Loss*, London, The Women's Press.

KALISH, R. A. (1985) *Death, Grief and Caring Relationships*, California, Brooks Cole.

KASTENBAUM, R. J. (1975) 'Is death a life Crisis? On the confrontation with death in theory and practice', in DATAN, M. and GINSBERG, L. H. (Eds) *Life-Span Developmental Psychology: Normative Life Crises*, New York, Academic Press.

KÜBLER-ROSS, E. (1969) *On Death and Dying*, New York, Macmillan.

LINDEMANN, E. (1944) 'Symptomatology and management of acute grief,' *American Journal of Psychiatry*, **101**, September, 141–8.

LITTLEWOOD, J. (1992a) *Aspects of Grief: Bereavement in Adult Life*, London, Routledge.

LITTLEWOOD, J. (1992b) 'On falling in love backwards', *Discussion Document*, Birmingham, National Association of Widows.

LITTLEWOOD, J. (1993a) 'A little widow is a dangerous thing: the amazing case of the women who simply refuse to disappear', keynote speech, *Annual General Meeting of the National Association of Widows*, Birmingham, National Association of Widows.

LITTLEWOOD, J. (1993b) 'The denial of death and rites of passage in contemporary societies,' in CLARK, D. (Ed.) *The Sociology of Death*, London, Blackwell.

MADDISON, D. and VIOLA, A. (1968) 'The health of widows in the year following bereavement', *Journal of Psychosomatic Research*, **12**, 297–3.

MARRIS, P. (1958) *Widows and their Families*, London, Routledge and Kegan Paul.

MARRIS, P. (1986) *Loss and Change* (2nd Edn) London, Routledge and Kegan Paul.

MORLEY, J. (1971) *Death, Heaven and the Victorians*, London, University of Pittsburgh Press.

MULKAY, M. (1993), 'Social death in Britain', in CLARK, D. (Ed.) *The Sociology of Death*, Oxford, Blackwell.

OAKLEY, A. (1979) 'Wisewomen and medicine man: changes in the management of childbirth', in MITCHELL, J. and OAKLEY, A. (Eds) *The Rights and Wrongs of Women*, Harmondsworth, Middlesex, Penguin Books.

OSTERWEISS, M., SOLOMON, F. and GREEN, M. (Eds) (1984) *Bereavement: Reactions, Consequences and Care*, Washington, DC, National Academy Press.

PARKES, C. (1972) *Bereavement*, New York, International Universities Press.

PARKES, C. (1975) 'What becomes of redundant world models? A contribution to the study of adaptation to change', *British Journal of Medical Psychology*, **48**, 131–7.

RAPHAEL, B. (1984) *The Anatomy of Bereavement: A Handbook for the Caring Professions*, London, Hutchinson.

ROWLAND, K.F. (1977) 'Environmental events predicting death for the elderly', *Psychological Bulletin*, **84**, 349–72.

WALTER, T. (1993) 'Sociologists never die: British Sociology and death', in CLARK, D. (Ed.) *The Sociology of Death*, Oxford, Blackwell.

WALVIN, J. (1986) 'Dying and mourning: the English case', in *Consequences of Mortality Trends and Differentials*, New York, United Nations.

YOUNG, M., BENJAMIN, B. and WALLACE, C. (1963) 'The mortality of widowers', *The Lancet*, **2**, 454–6.

Chapter 11

Feminist Reflections on the General Medical Council: Recreation and Retention of Male Power

Meg Stacey

During the Council debates on [presidential tenure] I noticed future presidents were always referred to as 'he'. When I rose to ask, for information, whether a woman could be a president, the entire Council collapsed in spontaneous laughter. When this finally subsided, the president assured me that she could be (Stacey, 1992, p. 94).

Understanding the Holders of Formal Power

Understandably, much feminist research has been about women, where we are, how we have been and are oppressed, how we have struggled to achieve greater space for our lives. This is understandable because women had been 'hidden from history' and overlooked — or looked down upon — in much research; understandable also because each of us works from the position we are in as to the kind of work we find it important for us to do. Furthermore, it is easier to research people like us — how can we, as women, know what it is to be a man? Then there are the problems about how to enter the men's world and about what we face if and when we do. In addition, the relatively powerless — women or men — are easier to research than the powerful; and, indeed, much mainstream (malestream) sociology has done just that.

However, no understanding of society can be complete without understanding of those who hold formal power as well as those who do not. This understanding is needed to achieve 'a sociology for rather than about women' (Olesen, 1994, p. 169). This includes understanding how the powerless can challenge, impede, perhaps overthrow the power-holders, or alternatively refrain from action (Kathy Davis' application of Giddens' conception of power to gender relations (Davis, 1988, 1991, ch. 4) is particularly interesting in this respect). Such understanding is necessary not only for completeness of academic knowledge, but also in order to develop strategies for effective action. Membership of the General Medical Council (GMC) — from 1976 to 1983 — opened a door into the male world. The GMC is a small segment of those with statutory power — the world of the regulators of British medicine, a largely male and certainly male-dominated domain.

Researchers, when writing up or discussing their work, usually state their theoretical position and also, especially when they have done field work using themselves overtly as research tools, explain something of their background and the role they played in the field in order to help readers assess the quality of their work and the inferences they make. This is the more important in this case because I changed role from member to researcher after my term of office on the GMC had finished. The resulting methodological problems I have discussed elsewhere (Stacey, 1994a). I did not accept appointment deliberately to do feminist research or any kind of research at all: that decision came later. I accepted, although I would have preferred to work on a policy-making body, in the spirit of public service.

How I Came To Be on the GMC

As a mother of young children I was upset about the stressful conditions in which children were nursed in hospitals in the 1960s, and became involved in both a pressure group and research about the care of children in hospital (Stacey, 1970; Hall and Stacey, 1979). This activity ultimately led to membership of the Welsh Hospital Board (WHB) from whence I was nominated to the Michael Davies committee on hospital complaints procedures. I suppose it was from such activities that my name 'emerged' and the Privy Council nominated me to the GMC.

The Men's World and the New Feminist Challenge

When I was appointed in 1976, my feminist thinking was undergoing much challenge and change. These derived partly from the impact of having been appointed two years previously to a British university chair

— the first woman to be so appointed at Warwick University — and partly from the impact of the Women's Liberation Movement (WLM). I have written briefly about the more personal parts of the WLM impact (Stacey, 1989), recording how I had felt excluded, belonging as I did to what I heard younger women calling the 'traitor generation' — those of us who had married, as I had, and became homemakers in the 1950s. However, at a personal level 'the most important and unexpected outcome for me of the WLM' was discovering I would be happier as a lesbian (Stacey, 1989, p. 140), a process which was emerging into consciousness during the last half of my time at the GMC.

Being simultaneously exposed in this way to masculinist power in the university, on the one hand, and the ebullient vision and demands of younger women, on the other, deepened and strengthened my understanding of feminism. Experience in the 'men's world' was radicalizing. Influenced by Juliet Mitchell's *Women's Estate* (1971) and bothered because, even before I came to Warwick, I had already been getting the tag of 'exceptional woman', I determined to reject the implied role. I knew that it had been fortunate circumstances, among them the explosion of sociology in the 1960s, which had led me to where I was. My life path was initially predicated on an earlier form of feminism absorbed from my suffragist mother and suffragette father. Starting with an education my parents selected as being 'as good as a boy's', the goal became to do the things that men do, which meant entering social spaces men had for centuries claimed for themselves. Not that I remember ever wanting to be a man; I was after the freedom to do things men did in the visible social world.

Developing Feminist Theoretical Critiques

Much was burgeoning in feminist academia in the 1970s. During my GMC membership, Marion Price and I wrote *Women, Power and Politics* (1981), which centres around the relative under-representation of women in the public domain. Other on-going work (with a group of Warwick researchers) on the division of labour in health care showed clearly the inadequacies of malestream theories of the professions, first expressed in the 'Two Adams' paper (Stacey, 1981) where I argued that all sociological theory hitherto had been developed by men to deal with public domain problems. The primarily domestic domain where women laboured was not included in this approach. The 'family', when mentioned by the founding fathers, was seen as rather curiously detached from society, and its later study as a somewhat second-rate sub-discipline.

Malestream theory offered little help in understanding the health professions, hospitals and clinics which had developed in the public domain but had incorporated social values and statuses from the domestic domain, most notable in the subordination of nurses (Gamarnikow, 1978). A new concept of 'intermediate domain' — intermediate that is between public and domestic — seemed necessary to handle this phenomenon (Stacey and Davies, 1983).

Drawing together feminist and malestream work for my book, *The Sociology of Health and Healing* (1988), advanced understanding of the relationship between the gender order and the health care division of labour. It showed how medicine had claimed high status for itself, subordinating occupations such as nursing and midwifery, filled largely or entirely by women. Historically, the GMC had played an important part in this. Theoretically it also became clear that the health care division of labour could not be properly understood or analyzed unless one included along with the paid health workers, the unpaid labourers, more often called 'carers', who are largely but not exclusively women.

By the time I came to write *Regulating British Medicine* (1992), much had been written about specific aspects of the division of labour in health care (notably Oakley, 1976; Gamarnikow, 1978; Graham, 1979, 1984; Finch and Groves, 1982). The essays *In a Man's World* (Spencer and Podmore, 1987) were revealing about divisions of labour between professional women and men. Empirical work from the USA on nursing (Olesen and Whittaker, 1968; Lewin and Olesen, 1981) and on the women's health movement and the professionalization of medicine (Ruzek, 1978) had challenged received thinking.

However, there was no extended theoretical feminist critique of the masculinism of sociological theories of the professions. Anne Witz had not yet published *Professions and Patriarchy* (1992) which treats extensively and valuably the struggles of women's occupations to gain professional status, but remains within the malestream tradition in that the old public domain concepts are used as tools of analysis, the importance of the unpaid health worker is ignored as is the crucial interface between public and private domains (see Gamarnikow, 1992, Stacey, 1993). Nor was there much work on 'race' and the health professions, a gap which Porter (1993) has begun to fill, as has Moss (1992).

Given the inadequacies of malestream theory, and faced with analyzing the male world of the GMC, Dorothy Smith's work, notably

The Everyday World as Problematic (1987), was especially helpful. With her I share theoretical assumptions about the importance of structure, and the crucial need to add gender to the traditional analyses of class and status. The way in which these abstract structural relations are experienced in the living social world, and how the interactions taking place there recreate and sustain those structures, fascinates me as it obviously does Dorothy Smith. Sitting on the GMC gave me an opportunity to examine one corner of that process at first hand. With hindsight I would say that my stance in writing about the GMC was similar to that of Porter, who says that the point of ethnography is not idiographically to illumine small scale events, 'but to use examination of human agency to shed light on the relationship between agency and structure' (Porter, 1993, p. 593).

Starting Points

Entering the GMC in 1967, I had a lively appreciation of the under-representation of women in public domain hierarchies, and a sensitive awareness of our oppression. Derived from personal experience and from empirical and theoretical academic work, I approached the GMC as a dedicated feminist with considerable experience in male-dominated hierarchies. I believed (and still do) in the equal worth of all human beings and remain an unreconstructed universalist in the sense that I believe in the availability of health and welfare services to all as basic citizen's rights. These views do not imply mechanical equalities but are about transcendental values which lead me to be uncomfortable with elitism. Connected with these notions, much of my academic work has been 'sociology for use', or applied sociology if you will.

My aim in writing *Regulating British Medicine* was to expose the pro-professional — and also masculinist and racist — characteristics of the GMC, hoping thereby to encourage practitioners to see what I believed I saw: namely, that although the members were well-meaning, hard-working people (mostly men) who sincerely believed they were doing a good job, in practice they were not adequately fulfilling their statutory function of protecting the public. I also wanted to make knowledge about that mystifying body available to the interested public, policy makers and pressure groups. In this chapter I shall expand the message by discussing the GMC from a feminist point of view.

The Constitution and Functions of the GMC

What was — and is — this body with which I had agreed to work? The GMC is a statutory body originally set up in 1858 and currently governed by the Medical Act of 1983. Independent of the state, it is financed by the profession whose registration fees and annual retention fees (which may be claimed as expenses for tax purposes) constitute a main source of income. Other sources are the fees charged for certain services. The Chief Medical Officer (CMO) of England (a civil servant) is always a Council member; the CMOs of Scotland, Wales and Northern Ireland have since 1979 sat in rotation, although in November, 1993, it was announced that all four CMOs would in future come to all meetings. After the 1978 Medical Act none of the CMOs was permitted to serve on any GMC committee: the profession's leaders guard its independence of the state jealously.

The essence of the GMC's powers, which are granted by Parliament, is its control of the registers of practitioners, which it keeps and publishes. The GMC controls entry to the registers by deciding what qualifications are necessary for registration. It does this by approving medical schools whose training and education are sufficiently in line with the guidance it offers as to the content of basic medical education. The guidance is established after thorough consultation with the medical schools and is not proscriptive; experimentation is encouraged. The Council may visit and inspect medical schools. Radically new guidance — *Tomorrow's Doctors* — was published in December, 1993: it remains to be seen how closely it will be implemented.

The GMC may remove from the register, temporarily or permanently, persons it considers have become unfit to practice. The GMC has no inspectorate, so relies on the reports of convictions or complaints made against practitioners to check on continuing competence to practise. If unfitness to practise seems to result from ill health, practitioners are dealt with under specific health procedures; 'ill health' is most often addiction to drink or drugs — occasionally an unrecognized incapacitating physical illness and also, rarely, homosexual relations with patients seen as a case for treatment rather than misconduct — the last, if 'serious' and including heterosexual misconduct, would lead practitioners to the conduct, not the health, committee.

Members of the GMC are drawn from three main sources: appointment by universities and royal colleges; election by registered medical practitioners of each of the four countries of the UK; and

Table 11.1   Mode of membership of Council Members; 1976, 1979, 1984 and 1993

	1976	1979	1984	1993
Appointed by				
Universities	18	21	21	21
Royal Colleges[1]	9	13	13	15
Total appointed	27	34	34	36
Elected by registered medical practitioners in				
England & Wales[2]	8			
England[2]		39	39	38
Scotland	2	6	6	7
Wales		3	3	3
Ireland	1			
Northern Ireland		2	2	2
Total elected	11	50	50	50
Nominated by Privy Council				
Medical	5	2	2	2
Non-medical	3	7[3]	9[3]	11[4]
Total nominated	8	9	11	13
Total Members	46	93	95	99

1. Royal Colleges include faculties and societies.
2. England includes the Channel Islands and the Isle of Man.
3. Includes one nurse.
4. Includes one nurse and one pharmacist.
Sources: GMC Minutes and Annual Reports, 1976, 1979, 1984, 1985; personal communication from GMC, 1990; Stacey, 1992.

nomination by the Queen in Privy Council (which rather mystifying term really means — in this context — by the Health Ministers). When I was first appointed, Council had forty-six members; in 1994 there are ninety-nine. Table 11.1 shows the modes of membership of the Council in 1976 when I joined, in 1979 after the 1978 Medical Act, in 1984, the year after I was replaced and in 1993.

Since 1979, elected members have a constitutional majority over all other members taken together. This is a prime route for rank and file doctors, particularly general practitioners (GPs), to gain a voice, but also a means whereby the British Medical Association (BMA) — the doctors' major trade union — can influence GMC policy and practice. The Privy Council nominees offer the state, in this case the government in power, some influence. Until 1926, when the first layman [*sic*] was appointed, all these state nominees were medical. The GMC now wishes the proportion of the lay to rise to a fifth by reducing the appointed members from the royal colleges.

The Registers

On the *main register* (or principal list) are recorded those doctors granted *full registration*. British-educated doctors who have satisfactorily completed their medical school qualifying examinations are admitted to the *provisional register* while they undertake their pre-registration year. Satisfactory completion of this admits them to full registration.

Doctors who qualify in *recognized* medical schools overseas are accepted for *full registration* so long as they have verified clinical experience not less extensive than they would have gained in the UK-pre-registration year. Those who lack this can apply for *provisional registration* and are only able to work in hospital house officer posts under supervision.

Traditions of Prejudice

Restriction of entry is of the essence in occupations claiming to be professions. Sometimes restriction is exercised not only against those lacking appropriate qualifications, but by using other considerations — such as 'inappropriateness'. The British register was used for many years to keep women out of medicine — how inappropriate for a woman to be a doctor! The particular arrangements for the admission of doctors from the former British empire, mentioned briefly above, are exposed in my book (Stacey, 1992, chs. 10 and 12). Not only ex-colonials but members of other nations experience this exclusivity: the GMC treated medical refugees from Nazi Germany less than generously and, more recently, tried but failed to control the free movement of European doctors into the UK (Stacey, 1994b).

Women and the GMC

Historical Background

Jean Scott (1984) — herself a one-time GMC member — has researched the GMC's reluctance to admit women to the medical register, a story which, in outline, is well known among feminists. The GMC, as established in 1858, was an entirely male body, drawn from medical schools and royal colleges. Elizabeth Blackwell, with medical qualifications from America, and having practised briefly in England before the Act was passed, early applied for admission to the register — which the Council found they had to grant. However, the Council soon blocked that route, invoking national boundaries and barring foreign qualifications. Elizabeth Garrett Anderson found another way; she became a nurse, took private tuition and sat the examination of the Royal Society of Apothecaries. That route the GMC also blocked.

The conflicting responsibilities of the powerful lead to internal contradictions which provide chinks and cracks through which the excluded may ultimately find a way (Davis, 1991, p. 73). So it was with the GMC. Aspiring women doctors had (male) friends in the House of Commons who pressed their cause against the intransigence of the medical schools and the GMC. In 1875, triggered by a Bill to permit the recognition of foreign medical degrees held by women, the Privy Council sought the (then) General Council of Medical Education's opinion about women and medicine. It concluded:

> The Council are of the opinion that the study and practice of medicine and surgery instead of affording a field of exertion well fitted for women, present special difficulties which cannot safely be ignored...but the Council are not prepared to say that women ought to be excluded (Quoted in Scott, 1984, p. 1766).

The concern that legislation should not interfere with academic freedom overrode objections to women entering medicine. If they were to be admitted, Council said their education and examination should be conducted entirely apart from men. Medical men were by no means converted. In 1876, three women applied to the Royal College of Surgeons of England to sit the diploma in midwifery, possession of which entitled the holder to registration. Lawyers informed the college that it had to admit them: the examiners promptly resigned.

Women Enter Medicine

Change was slow. Most medical schools continued to be reluctant to admit women. Ninety years later, the Royal Commission on Medical Education of 1965–68 (the Todd Report) (Todd, 1968) reported that 'women candidates often have special difficulty in gaining admission to medical schools' (para. 301). It reminded its readers that, more than twenty years before, the Goodenough Committee (Goodenough, 1944) had recommended that 'a substantial proportion of all medical schools, perhaps a fifth, should be for women' and that shortly afterwards the (then) University Grants Committee stipulated that the proportion should normally not fall below 15 per cent. When Todd was sitting, with the unique exception of the Royal Free Hospital where about a half of the students were women, the proportion of women medical students was about 24 per cent. The proportion varied, the Royal Free apart, from 35 per cent at Leeds to 11 per cent at the London (see also Todd, 1968, Table 7, Appendix 9).

Data from an ASME (Association for the Advancement of Medical Education) survey (Todd, 1968, Appendix 19) suggested medical schools applied more stringent criteria to women than to men, and often judged women applicants irrationally, with the result that outstanding women candidates were sometimes rejected. Headmistresses believed that their teachers discouraged many of their best pupils from applying for medicine.

The Commission's view was that since some medical schools admitted a high proportion of women their presence raised 'few or no serious problems' (para. 302). Available evidence led it to believe that there was a higher wastage rate among women (but see Elston, 1977, 1980) and so it thought that a shortage of medical school places might justify preference for men. Nevertheless, it concluded:

> the main criteria for admission to a medical course should be the ability of the applicant to profit from the course and to become a good doctor. Moreover, medicine demands and deserves the best recruits it can get, irrespective of their sex (Todd, 1968, para. 303).

Medical Women's Careers

Medical schools abolished the quota system after the Sex Discrimination Act, 1975. However, Isobel Allen's (1988) evidence suggested that while the proportion of women medical students was approaching 50 per cent, *de facto* discrimination against women had simply moved up the career ladder. She had interviewed (spring, 1986) 314 men and 326 women spread over three cohorts, qualifying in 1966, 1976 and 1981 respectively, with average ages of 43, 33 and 28. Women's and men's careers could be compared, the women's careers contextualised and, by inference, changes in medicine also noted.

Some interesting career differences emerged. Ninety-five per cent of the men compared with 56 per cent of the women were working full-time; 2 per cent of the men and 36 per cent of the women were working less than full-time. About 5 per cent of the women were not working at the time of interview, but most of these had worked in medicine for some years after qualification and while they had small children — most intended to return to medicine. Some clear specialty differences emerged. General practice was fairly evenly divided (39 per cent of men; 36 per cent of women); more men (57 per cent) than women (46 per cent) were in hospital medicine; but many fewer men (1 per cent) than women (11 per cent) were in community medicine.

A striking finding was that while 17 per cent of men were consultants, only 10 per cent of women had achieved that status — although roughly equal proportions of men and women were registrars, senior registrars and senior house officers. Thirty-two per cent of the men compared with 23 per cent of the women were GP principals. Principals and consultants are the two categories in which doctors may practice independently. All others are subordinate in some way. Nearly twice as many men as women were in academic medicine. On the other hand, the 'overwhelming majority' of clinical assistants and associate specialists (which are not career grades) and all but one of the senior clinical medical officers and clinical medical officers (also not career grades) were women. Men also did more private work than women (Allen, 1988, pp. 324–25).

The impact of the domestic domain differed for men and women. Women put off having children for longer than men.

> Both men and women agreed that women needed to plan ahead and needed help in succeeding in a career structure which was essentially geared to the full-time commitment of ambitious and single-minded men who are able to ignore domestic commitments (Allen, 1988, p. 326).

Staff in medical school were believed by both men and women to treat women students differently from men, while in hospital training, consultants' discriminatory treatment was particularly commented upon.

> Some teaching staff were said not to rate women highly and to assume they were not career-minded, as well as making sexist remarks, putting women into humiliating situations and making statements which could only be regarded as derogatory. This kind of treatment was thought to put women off hospital medicine, and discourage them from surgery in particular (Allen, 1988, p. 326).

The Department of Health working party which followed these revelations focused on the under-representation of women at consultant level; opportunities for part-time working; and equal opportunities in appointment procedures. Its own 1989 evidence confirmed the Allen findings. Women in general had been shown to be no less able and committed to medical careers than men, but, taking all medical specialties together, only 15 per cent of consultants were women and striking differences between specialties remained. Thirteen per cent of consultants in the general medical specialties were women, but only 3 per cent in surgical specialties; nearly 20 per cent in anaesthetics and over 20 per cent of consultants in radiology, pathology and psychiatry. The working party made detailed recommendations to overcome this situation, contrary as it is to law on sex equality, and wasteful of national investment in medical training (DH, 1991).

Women on the GMC

For women to be registered as medical practitioners is, of course, quite another thing from membership of the GMC. In response to the unequal treatment of women doctors in the armed forces in the First World War, the Medical Women's Federation was founded in 1917 with the specific aim of working for equal treatment with men (Scott, 1988). In 1924, the Federation resolved to get women onto the GMC. Progress was slow: Christine Murrell was elected in 1933, but died before she could take her seat. Subsequent attempts all failed until 1955 when Dr Janet Aitkin was elected, although the Privy Council had nominated the Rt. Hon. Florence Horsburgh in 1950.

Women are still under-represented on the GMC, but things are improving. In 1976, when I was first appointed, there were only three women (two lay; one elected doctor) out of a total of forty-six members. Since the Council was reformed and enlarged in 1979, the number and the proportion have slowly increased. That year there were eight women out of a Council of ninety-three; five were elected out of the total of fifty elected doctors; the three others were lay members appointed by the Privy Council.

In 1994, ten elected women doctors were sitting and a further one was nominated by a royal college. The total remained less than their proportion on the register where in 1991 nearly 38 per cent were women. The Chief Medical Officer for Wales (whose turn it was) in 1994 is a woman. There were in addition three lay women appointed, one of whom was also a member of an ethnic minority. She has double minority status within the Council, being neither white nor male.

In 1976, no doctors had come from ethnic minorities, in 1979 six were elected from the nominees of the Overseas Doctors Association (ODA) — all men — but in 1994, of the overseas doctors elected, five were men and one a woman.

The Masculinist Ethos

I was not the only woman who felt she had strayed into a gentleman's club. The Council retained this ethos in the mid-1970s and into the 1980s. From the gallery it appears much the same in the 1990s, except of course there are more women, more of whom are radical or reformist. Outside the council chamber, before and after sessions, they seem able quite openly to form groups to discuss their common interests, whether as doctors or as GMC members. In 1979, the big change had been that there were now enough of us to exchange ideas when we met in the loo during breaks in meetings. (The only women's toilets were either in the basement or the attic — see also Barbara Wootton's (1967) hilarious accounts of her problems with such accommodation when she first entered the male world of government office earlier this century.)

A main objective when the Council was founded was to convince 'the public' (that is, men) that they could trust registered medical practitioners to treat them appropriately, including entrusting their wives to their care. An objective of the medical profession, and one which the GMC helped greatly to fulfil, was to achieve the upward mobility of medical practitioners so that they might be accepted as 'gentlemen' and, when making house calls, be admitted through the front door rather than the tradesman's entrance. How the profession succeeded in improving the material rewards and the status of doctors has been well documented. It was greatly aided by alliance with the rising bourgeoisie and the enrolment of their wives as patients (Parry and Parry, 1976; Inkster, 1977; Waddington, 1984; Davidoff and Hall, 1987, pp. 308–10 and 338–40). The London club atmosphere of the GMC was one way in which the claims to gentlemanly status could be asserted both symbolically and materially in terms of style and standard of services available.

The quotation at the head of this chapter vividly conveys the continued masculinism of the Council. I was sure at the time the laughter was mostly about the ludicrousness of thinking of a woman president. There are, of course, other possible explanations. My point of order was an interruption in a serious and anxiety-making debate about limiting the term of the presidency. This limitation, strongly desired by many and finally agreed, related to Council's wish to be able in future to vote for a youngish president (that is, a person in his (sic) fifties rather than sixties) without the risk of having a president in office for decades, as had occurred in the past. Perhaps my interruption just released the tension. I remain convinced it was more than that.

The hilarity which greeted my question (it was 1981) and the president's prompt and utterly correct reply showed the difference between the formal equal rights of all members and the social reality of the plausibility of those rights being fully accorded. Dame Josephine Barnes had been President of the Royal Society of Medicine and of the Council of the BMA before that. Dame Annis Gillie was President of the Royal College of General Practitioners as long ago as 1964–67, but there has been no woman president since. Professor Dame Barbara Clayton had yet to become President of the Royal College of Pathologists (1984–87) and Dame Margaret Turner-Warwick of the Royal College of Physicians of London (1989–1992). Fiona Caldecott is currently (1994) President of the Royal College of Psychiatrists. Neither the Surgeons nor the Obstetricians and Gynaecologists have yet elected a woman president. These exceptions confirm that women can hold high medical office, but those who do still count as 'exceptional women'. At the time of the laughter episode all chairpersons of GMC committees were men and hence all those on the dais at formal meetings were men. It would be from among those that a president would be normally elected. In 1994, a woman will be a treasurer, the first one ever.

That women were accepted if we kept our place (allocated by men) was my impression. Undoubtedly, the president meant to be friendly, supportive and to ease my path when he introduced me the first day I arrived by saying (according to my diary).

> I had a remarkable career, was a full professor in my own right, had achieved a situation in which my husband also had a chair, but he thought that in these days of equality I had put his career first. He added that the Council had not had a sociologist member before (27.5.76).

The message I heard was that although I was a woman — and despite the sociology — I might get by because I was seen to have been a dutiful wife.

Another aspect of the masculinist ethos relates to sexual relations between doctors and patients. Here the context of (male-led) discussion rested heavily on the great risks that doctors run at the hands of their women patients. Many times was I told, in a confidential tone of voice, the tale of the 'siren' who came into the surgery determined to have her practitioner lay her. These tales had a myth-like character, a folk tale, what Malinowski understands as a 'charter for action'. Faced with this body of 'knowledge' I found myself unable to convey to the medical men my own empirical knowledge that many women experience unwanted minor, and sometimes not so minor, sexual advances. The 'action' the tale sanctioned was to be forgiving to men practitioners who succumbed to this overwhelmingly powerful temptation to which they were subjected. Again, a crack in the hegemony emerges: American medical speakers have warned the profession that it is essential to take sexual abuse of patients more seriously, for their research has shown that it is all too common and, what is more, women are ceasing to stand for it (Stacey, 1992, pp. 225–26; Fisher and Fahy, 1990).

Great courtesy was extended to women, to GMC lay members and to overseas doctors. But, as a senior member of their number pointed out to me, the courtesies served only to emphasise our otherness. As I wrote:

> Like women, overseas doctors were often invited to sit with the president during lunches being taken between sessions: civilly treated, well looked after, but kept in their place, in fact gently and unobtrusively patronized (Stacey, 1992, p. 209).

I have no doubt the intentions in inviting us 'others' to sit with them was done by successive presidents with the best of intentions. That non-whites and women could experience it as patronizing derives from the pervasive exclusivist attitudes. I do not recall such invitations emerging at 'official functions'; the president's right and left hands would then be graced by people whose status, office or relationship commanded it.

Other actions were more genuinely welcoming. Two medical men nominated me, for example, to be a fellow (sic) of the Royal Society of Medicine. Ironically, this 'patronage' did not feel patronizing. My academic merit and my status as a Council member justified such nomination, as it were 'of right'. Contradictions of this kind I shall return to, for they are the essence of the internal contradictions which make change, including in places of power, possible.

As I argued in my book, and argue here, specifically in relation to women, what happens at the GMC is the result of historical legacy. However, what happens in the present is also the result of how members are reacting to the changes and challenges in the present world around them. As I wrote — and as remains true:

> Women students and women junior hospital doctors now constitute a 'critical mass' and so can support each other and retain their identity as women. Change will be slow, as it always is in any time or place where the ceding or sharing of power is in question. The changes have not yet worked through to the elite level of medicine and only in the last five years have they even begun to be reflected in the Council (Stacey, 1992, pp. 207–8).

That a young woman doctor, newly elected, could suggest in its annual report that the GMC is seen as sexist and racist is change indeed (McCallum, 1989, p. 4).

Women are still less likely than men of similar medical standing to receive merit awards, additional payments above the scale rate, although possibly few of either sex appreciated that. Women were invisible to the 'old boy network' which had been screening out women without the men being aware of it. A senior male member when he learned that senior women on the GMC had not been given them was, as reported to me, appropriately surprised and even possibly dismayed. But it is precisely in those ways that men do act as a group to sustain their own power and privilege.

That people are not always aware of what they are doing, and of how the institutions of which they are a part continually support and maintain particular dominant norms and values, is a well-understood sociological phenomenon. The characteristics of medicine as an exclusive and fiercely cohesive collectivity undoubtedly exaggerate this tendency. Relevant here is what Vogel describes as the often-observed capacity of patriarchal power for self-mystification (Vogel, 1988, p. 145). Vogel speaks also of the 'blurred distinction between the dimensions of power and protection in the [civil] law's discriminatory treatment of women', which she says 'must be taken as the characteristic of the unique feature of their "oppression", compared with the condition of other under-privileged groups' (Vogel, 1988, p. 143).

This blurring, deriving from the perception of women primarily as sexual objects and child-bearers, was apparent in GMC discussions about women. Senior members took it for granted that a woman would not have a career such as a man might have; they would marry, bear and rear children. When issues around job-sharing arose there was sympathy expressed (from the dais itself), because it would 'help women' as well as avoiding wastage of highly and expensively trained medical personnel.

Never did I hear it mentioned that a man who wished to share child rearing and domesticity with his partner might be similarly helped. Cowardly perhaps, I never challenged that particular masculinist assumption, as I did many others. I suppose I judged that what I said would be so little understood that it would be a waste of time, indeed, perhaps even counter-productive. This may be an example of when I may have behaved differently because I was attending the meetings as a political being and not as a researcher, let alone a feminist one; in the latter case I should have raised the question to uncover an unspoken norm whose existence I could only infer.

This assumption of women's different life path, not only because of the biology of reproduction but because of the social arrangements which have traditionally surrounded child-rearing, is also found in Allen's (1988) account of doctors' careers. Indeed, it permeates the recommendations both of her study and that of the Department of Health working party (1991). It supports my argument that a feminist theory of the professions has to take account of the heterosexual domestic domain and norms surrounding it as well as women's activity in the public domain.

What GMC Women Thought about Their Status

Medical women who had come up through the system and reached the GMC had a variety of responses to the place they had been accorded in the medical gender order. Some were 'honorary males'. One university woman who had been appointed turned away when I congratulated her on her achievement as a woman. Such women had got by, and got on, by suppressing — indeed denying — the relevance, both to themselves and others, of all the differences between themselves and the men. One not only denied she had ever been the victim of discrimination but appeared to deny it existed at all — doctors were doctors, all equal and apparently genderless.

In understanding the stance of such women I find helpful Komter's (1991, pp. 57ff) discussion of Gramsci's (1971) concept of ideological hegemony applied to the context of power and gender. This is the consensus expressed by subordinate groups in approval of the dominant values, symbols, beliefs and opinions. While appearing to derive from free will, such stances reflect necessities which stem from existing relations of dominance. But not all who are unaware of gender oppression necessarily accepted all facets of the medical establishment's hegemony. One, for example, had been a leading activist in the professional revolt against the GMC in the late sixties (see Stacey, 1992, ch. 4).

Other women members are highly conscious of the disadvantages under which women labour. Some are active in the Medical Women's Federation, still working in a style which could be said to follow a model more common earlier this century before the WLM. At least two others are more radical and work through and with more recent feminist organizations such as Women into Medicine (WIM). All (except the extreme examples of 'honorary males') had a sense of, and articulated, the commonality of women and their experiences of problems as being different from those of men.

Medicine or Gender?

The president's response to my question about whether a woman could be a president shows, as I said, a division between men behaving as men — with unspoken assumptions about the proper ordering of the world — and their understanding of principles of equal citizenship and of equality within medicine. The GMC has always sustained the notion (however fictional) that all registered medical practitioners are equal. This was a crucial element in the successful professionalization of the occupation of medicine, making the unity of the profession possible. Without that continued unity which the GMC has promoted, it would lose its legitimacy to regulate medicine. This leads to an imperative that rules must apply equally to all. The profession of medicine has, after all, even if belatedly and under duress, accepted women as members.

A distinction between being a woman and being a doctor also emerged, especially in discussion with this lay woman when she represented a non-medical perspective on a common problem. Sometimes, the discourse of womanhood was paramount and the injustices of a male world were evoked by feminists of all kinds. However, in the middle of such a discussion a challenge to medicine would at once evoke the discourse of medicine, turning 'women' immediately into 'medical scientists' or 'medical practitioners' who, as doctors, had a strong commonality with the medical men they had just been blaming.

This seems somewhat more complicated than a minority group simply taking on the ideology of a dominant group, or exerting their agency although accepting their inferiority. Despite their subordinate position in the gender order (which some would insist is not subordinate but complementary) these women are themselves members of the dominant medical group. Their livelihood and a good deal about the way they think of the world derives from their medical training: this they share with their male colleagues.

The GMC, furthermore, represents an arena in which women join with men in the exertion of power. The women, along with the men, make decisions which affect the lives and earning ability of men as well as women. A few of them are acutely aware of how the effects of the gender order of our society as a whole are embroiled in those decisions in ways it may not always be easy to tease out — the masculinism which underlies much obstetric practice, for example. Despite large areas of mutuality of purpose and action, in which women share the exercise of power with men, the GMC remains an arena in which the subordination of women is visible, if not always recognized.

This is not surprising, for if men continue to act as a group to retain their power and privileges in public and domestic domains alike, one would expect that the more the power, the higher the office, the more tenacious the men are likely to be. The GMC provided me with a good lesson in how subtly (and even unconsciously) such power is exercised. It also provided a lesson in internal contradictions within the ambitions and actions of the group and how this has led, and will continue to lead, the men to many compromises.

What of the Future?

The GMC is under immense pressure to bring its regulatory practices into the modern world; it has lost its unchallenged superiority — along with medicine generally and all other professions. Government is critical of its performance on a number of matters, and has for two years failed to find parliamentary time to increase the GMC's powers to discipline under-performing doctors. Government has set up its own enquiry about this so far as the NHS is concerned — and this in addition to enquiries about specialist education and the NHS complaints procedures, both of which impinge on the GMC. The editor of the *British Medical Journal* fears it is being side-lined (Smith, 1993). Patients' pressure groups are generally dissatisfied with the way the GMC handles their complaints; and lay women's groups are pressing on issues such as abuse of women patients by their doctors which the Council has traditionally not pursued as rigorously as it should.

hese tensions constitute the 'chinks and cracks' which make space for oppressed groups to effect change. It seems likely that the GMC will have to be transformed if it is to survive at all. Part of that transformation, if the medical women are strong enough — and the proportion they constitute of the profession is still increasing — will inevitably include a reduction in, and ultimate removal of, the masculinist ethos. However, one should not underestimate the power of male elite groups to survive. Their prestige — and the home comfort of many of them — is linked to the *status quo*. Progressive GMC women and their male allies will have to work hard to abolish the masculinist ethos, which is part of the wider ethos which makes the GMC look increasingly inappropriate in the modern world.

Nevertheless, the process of change will be slow; as I remarked of the 1970s and 1980s, life:

> on the Council was not entirely nineteenth century... the founding fathers would have felt out of place in a number of ways. But given their pervasive legacy, they would have felt happier there than in many parts of the outside world (Stacey, 1992, pp. 204–5).

In the 1990s, I suspect this is still true, but marginally less so.

References

ALLEN, I. (1988) *Doctors and their Careers*, London, Policy Studies Institute.

DAVIDOFF, L. and HALL, C. (1987) *Family Fortunes: Men and Women of the English Middle Class 1780–1850*, London, Hutchinson.

DAVIS, K. (1991) 'Critical sociology and gender relations', in DAVIES, K., LEIJENAAR, M. and OLDERSMA, J. (Eds) *The Gender of Power*, London, Sage, pp. 65–86.

DEPARTMENT OF HEALTH (1991) *Women Doctors and their Careers. Report of the Joint Working Party*, London, Department of Health.

ELSTON, M. A. (1977) 'Women in the medical profession: whose problem?', in STACEY, M., REID, M., HEATH, C. and DINGWALL, R. (Eds) *Health and the Division of Labour*, London, Croom Helm, pp. 115–40.

ELSTON, M. A. (1980) 'Medicine', in SILVERSTON, R. and WARD, A. (Eds) *Careers of Professional Women*, London, Croom Helm, pp. 99–139.

FINCH, J. and GROVES, D. (1982) *A Labour of Love: Women, Work and Caring*, London, Routledge and Kegan Paul.

FISHER, N. and FAHY, T. (1990) 'Sexual relations between doctors and patients', *Journal of the Royal Society of Medicine*, **83**, 681–83.

GAMARNIKOV, E. (1978) 'Sexual divisions of labour: the case of nursing', in KUHN, A., and WOLPE, A. M. (Eds) *Feminism and Materialism*, London, Routledge and Kegan Paul, pp. 96–123.

GAMARNIKOV, E. (1992) Review of WITZ, A. *Professions and Patriarchy, Sociology of Health and Illness*, **14**(4), 531–33.

GOODENOUGH REPORT (1944) *Report of the Interdepartmental Committee on Medical Schools*, London, HMSO.

GRAHAM, H. (1979) ' "Prevention and Health: every mother's business": a comment on child health policy in the seventies', in HARRIS, C. (Ed.) *The Sociology of the Family: New directions for Britain*, Keele, University of Keele, *Sociological Review*, Monograph 28, 160–85.

HARRIS, C. (1984) *Women Health and the Family*, Brighton, Wheatsheaf (Harvester).

GRAMSCI, A. (1971) *Selections from the Prison Notebooks*, London, Lawrence and Wishart.

HALL, D. and STACEY, M. (Eds) (1979) *Beyond Separation: further studies of children in hospital*, London, Routledge and Kegan Paul.

KOMTER, A. (1991) 'Gender, power and feminist theory', in DAVIS, K., LEIJNAAR, M. and OLDERSMA, J. (Eds) *The Gender of Power*, London, Sage, 42–62.

McCALLUM, A. 'First Impressions', *GMC Annual Report for 1989*, London, GMC, pp. 4–5.

MERRISON REPORT (1975) *Report of the Committee of Inquiry Into the Regulation of the Medical Profession*, Cmnd, 6018, London, HMSO.

MITCHELL, J. (1971) *Woman's Estate*, Harmondsworth, Penguin.

MOSS, P. (1992) 'The Migration and Racialization of Doctors from the Indian Sub-continent' University of Warwick, Unpublished Ph.D. thesis.

OAKLEY, A. (1976) 'Wise women and medicine man: changes in the management of childbirth', in MITCHELL, J. and OAKLEY, A. (Eds) *The Rights and Wrongs of Women*, Harmondsworth, Penguin, pp. 17–58.

OLESEN, V. and WHITTAKER, E. (1968) *The Silent Dialogue: a study of the social psychology of professional socialization*, San Francisco, Jossey Bass.

PORTER, S. (1993) 'Critical realist ethnography: the case of racism and professionalism in a medical setting', *Sociology*, 27(4), 591–609.

RUZEK, S. R. (1978) *The Women's Health Movement: feminist alternatives to medical care*, New York, Praeger.

SCOTT, J. (1984) 'Women and the GMC', *British Medical Journal*, **298**, 1764–67.

SCOTT, J. (1988) 'Women and the GMC: the struggle for representation', *Journal of the Royal Society of Medicine*, **81**, 164–66.

SMITH, D. (1987) *The Everyday World as Problematic*, Milton Keynes, Open University Press.

SMITH, R. (1993) 'The end of the GMC?' *British Medical Journal*, **307**, 954.

SPENCER, A. and PODMORE, D. (1987) *In a Man's World: Essays on Women in Male-dominated Professions*, London, Tavistock.

STACEY, M. (Ed.) (1970) *Hospitals, Children and their Families*, London, Routledge and Kegan Paul.

STACEY, M. (1981) 'The division of labour revisited or overcoming the two Adams', in ABRAMS, P. and DEEM, R. (Eds) *Practice and Progress: British Sociology 1950–1980*, London, Allen and Unwin, pp. 172–90.

STACEY, M. (1988) *The Sociology og Health and Healing: a Textbook*, London, Unwin Hyman.

STACEY, M. (1989) 'A note about my experience of the WLM', *Feminist Review*, **31**, 140–42.

STACEY, M. (1992) *Regulating British Medicine: the General Medical Council*, London, Wylie.

STACEY, M. (1993) Review of WITZ, A. *Professions and Patriarchy, Sociology*, 27(3), 543–44.

STACEY, M. (1994a) 'From being a native to becoming a researcher', in BURGESS, R. G. (Ed.) *Issues in Qualitative Sociology*, London, JAI Press.

STACEY, M. and PRICE, M. (1981) *Women Power and Politics*, London, Tavistock.

STACEY, M. and DAVIES, C. (1983) *Division of Labour in Child Health Care: Final Report to the SSRC*, Coventry, University of Warwick.

TODD REPORT (1968) *Royal Commission on Medical Education 1965–68: Report*, Cmnd, 3569, London, HMSO.

VOGEL, U. (1988) 'Under permanent guardianship: women's condition under modern civil law', in JONES, K. B. and JONASDOTTIR, A. G. *The Political Interests of Gender*, London, Sage, pp. 135–59.

WADDINGTON, I. (1984) *The Medical Profession in the Industrial Revolution*, London, Croom Helm.

WILLIAMS, A. (1993) 'Diversity and agreement in feminist ethnography', *Sociology*, **27**(4), 575–89.

WITZ, A. (1992) *Professions and Patriarchy*, London, Routledge.

WOOTON, B. (1967) *In a World I Never Made: Autobiographical Reflections*, London, Allen and Unwin.

Notes on Contributors

Lesley Doyal is Professor of Health Studies at the University of the West of England, Bristol. She has published extensively on women's health issues and is joint editor (with Jennie Naidoo and Tamsin Wilton) of *AIDS: Setting a Feminist Agenda* (Falmer Press, 1994).

Elizabeth Ettorre was formerly at the Addiction Unit, Institute of Psychiatry, London, but now lives and works in Finland. Her publications include *Women and Substance Use* (Macmillan and Rutgers University Press, 1992).

Ellen M. Goudsmit was formerly based in the Department of Human Sciences, Brunel University, Uxbridge, Middlesex. She has a particular interest in the psychologisation of illness, and has published several articles on this topic.

Hilary Graham is Professor of Applied Social Studies at the University of Warwick, Coventry. Her research has focused on women's experiences of caring for children, and on the effects of poverty. Her most recent book is *Hardship and Health in Women's Lives* (Harvester Wheatsheaf, 1993).

Janet Holland is Senior Research Officer in the Social Science Research Unit, Institute of Education, University of London, and Lecturer in Education at the Open University. She is currently researching family interactional practices and is a contributor to the *Men, Risk and AIDS Project*.

Kate Hunt is based at the MRC Medical Sociology Unit, University of Glasgow. Her most recent research is on hormone replacement therapy, and she has published widely on this and other topics relating to women's health.

Celia Kitzinger is Director of Women's Studies at Loughborough University. She is co-author (with Rachel Perkins) of *Changing Our Minds: Lesbian Feminism and Psychology* (Onlywomen and New York University Press, 1993) and co-editor (with Sue Wilkinson) of *Heterosexuality: A 'Feminism & Psychology' Reader* (Sage Publications, 1993).

Jane Littlewood is a Senior Lecturer in Social Sciences, Loughborough University. She is researching in the area of death and dying, and is the author of *Aspects of Grief: Bereavement in Adult Life* (Routledge, 1992).

Pat Spallone is at the Centre for Women's Studies, University of York. Her particular interest is in reproductive technologies, and she is the author of *Generation Games: Genetic Engineering and the Future for Our Lives* (The Women's Press and Temple University Press, 1992).

Meg Stacey is Emeritus Professor in the Department of Sociology, University of Warwick, Coventry. Her many publications on health-related issues include *Changing Human Reproduction: Social Science Perspectives* (Sage Publications, 1992) and *Regulating British Medicine* (Wiley, 1992).

Rachel Thomson is Senior Development Officer for the Sex Education Forum at the National Children's Bureau. She is a contributor to the *Men, Risk and AIDS Project*, and her recent publications include a number of chapters in this area.

Rose Wiles is a Research Fellow at the Institute for Health Policy Studies, University of Southampton, where she has carried out research on private health care, counselling and healthy lifestyles, as well as on women and health. Her contribution to this volume is based on her doctoral thesis.

Sue Wilkinson is based in the Department of Social Sciences, Loughborough University, having begun her research on breast cancer while Senior Lecturer in Health Studies Research at the University of Hull. She is the founding, and current, Editor of *Feminism & Psychology: An International Journal*, and also edits the book series *Gender and Psychology: Feminist and Critical Perspectives* (both Sage Publications).

Index